ON BORROWED TIME

ON BORROWED TIME

CALEN TEMPLETON

Calen Templeton

These are my personal experiences.
and I have tried to represent events as faithfully as possible.
I have tried to share my honest feelings,
for better or worse.

Copyright © 2022 Calen Templeton

To request permissions, contact the publisher at
Crazycal179@sbcglobal.net

Paperback: 978-1-0879-5861-3

Cover Art: Kenny Peris
Layout/Cover Design/Editor: Emily Templeton

Contents

For Dad

If you know him, you know all the reasons why.
If you don't, by the end, you will.

I love you, dad. Thank you for everything.

June 1

I had been feeling terrible for a few months, but I kept pushing towards November first. I had recently started a new job and that was the day my health insurance would kick in. But if I'm being honest, I was holding out until my life insurance kicked in.

I really did feel like I was dying. I couldn't breathe and had to stop to catch my breath after walking just a few feet. Nighttime was the worst, laying down to sleep was impossible. I could hear fluid in my lungs as I tried to breath and woke up in a choking panic every hour.

Finally, my wife, Jeanette, had enough and insisted I schedule a doctor appointment. I went online and found my doctor had recently retired. I was starting fresh and picked the first available time slot, it was for mid-January.

"Are you crazy!? You can't wait three months!"

I checked a different hospital and set up an appointment for November third, two days after my new insurance was active.

Being a Wednesday, the only busy day each week at work, I asked my new boss if I could come in a little late. My appointment was for 7:30 and my workday started at 8:30.

I dragged myself out of bed much earlier than I was accustomed to waking up and made my way to the appointment. Sitting in the waiting room, it was getting to be much closer to eight o'clock and they still hadn't called me back. I thought about leaving and calling later to reschedule. The nurse finally took me back and started getting me checked in and checking my vitals.

"How much do you weigh?"

"165... But maybe we should check, just to be sure."

"Okay, hop on the scale." I did as I was told and climbed up. It was much more work than it should have been. Everything hurt at this point. But I had a feeling that my weight was not as simple as it usually was.

"Yeah, you're 192!" She told me, surprised. I was almost thirty pounds heavier than I had usually been.

The doctor called in to say she was caught in traffic and would be there shortly. I waited longer, starting to get very concerned that I would miss the entire first half of my workday. Again, contemplating leaving for work and coming another time. But I was in the little doctor's office now, I was going to stay and wait as long as I had to.

After another twenty minutes, the doctor finally came in. She put that little plastic clamp on my finger. I never knew what that thing did, apparently, it's to check your oxygen. And apparently mine was really low. I don't know if there is a general guideline that doctors follow that says they should avoid showing an "Oh shit! Face" when looking over new patients, but she couldn't help herself. I knew it wasn't good when she slowly excused herself from the room.

A few minutes later she returned, and we discussed how I had been feeling.

"I'm having a lot of trouble breathing."

"Yes, I had a hunch you were going to say that. You need to go to the hospital."

"Okay, well I need to get to work. It's a busy Wednesday, you know. I'll call and make an appointment for next week."

"You don't understand. I already called an ambulance for you. I'm amazed you were able to drive here without passing out and crashing your car."

That is when I knew things were serious. The ambulance arrived and they didn't even trust me to take the few steps out of the tiny office. There were four men, and they wheeled the stretcher in and secured me with straps and hooked me up to an oxygen tank. I was loaded into the ambulance and away we went to the hospital. I was able to finally text work that I might not be in by lunch, after all.

I was in the hospital for two weeks. They told me I had kidney failure and if I hadn't come in when I did, I'd be dead within the week. They performed an emergency surgery to insert a catheter into my chest. This was to start dialysis. I didn't even know what dialysis was, but I was going to learn fast.

They did emergency sessions on me over the first three days of my hospital stay. They removed two liters of fluid that my body had been holding each time for a total of six liters. Take a moment to visualize that, three two-liter bottles of pop swishing around. That would explain the thirty pounds I recently gained and the swelling in my legs that was so bad I was wearing shoes that were two sizes too big.

That was seven months ago. It is now June 2022. I'm doing much better and feeling pretty good. I'm looking to get back to work and I took on a 33 mile in thirty days challenge to raise money and awareness for the National Kidney Foundation.

I've decided to start a journal of sorts as my second book. Go order my first one, A Few Cards Short, on Amazon, or email me at CRAZYCAL179@SBCGLOBAL.NET for a copy. That one is much more lighthearted than this will be. I wrote it when I was in a much better place... And not dying.

I hope you get something out of this book. I don't know exactly where it's going to take me. I have a bunch of topics in mind to cover, but who knows where we will end up by the end.

June 2

Define your life with a single word.

.
.
.
.
.
.
.
.
.
.
.
.
.
.
.
.
.
.
.
.

It's a trick, of course, no one can be reduced to one solitary character trait, except maybe the shallowest characters in a poorly written movie. I used to feel the same way about myself... Family, work, friends. I played many different roles to many different people in my life.

They all came to a crashing halt on the morning of November 3, 2021. Since that day, I can easily define my life with a single word... It is literally keeping me alive, while also killing me at the same time.

Dialysis

Most people don't know what dialysis means, not really. I certainly didn't. I knew it was for old people and on TV (see the first season of B-Positive) they sit around, reading and chatting and being charming. I only ever knew one person on dialysis, a customer at GameStop would come in before his appointments for games and mention it briefly. He was pretty young, and I never got the full story of why he went so often.

Dialysis is the type of word that you hope to never know too much about. If you picked up this book to learn the fine details, you have come to the wrong place. There are plenty of numbers to keep track of. I have to keep my iron and calcium levels high enough and my phosphorous level low enough. The doctors go over my lab work once a month and I always hope for more smiley faces than frown faces.

The best way I can describe it is that a big machine sucks all your blood out of your body, cleans it, and then puts it back. That is how "in-center" hemo works. It is meant to replace the job your kidneys are supposed to be doing. But kidneys are cleaning the blood twenty-four hours a day, dialysis is generally three times a week. Mine was every other day from 10 a.m. until 3 in the afternoon.

Everyone was commenting on all the time I'd have to read or watch movies. But what no one understands is how painful and draining it is. I would get such bad headaches and my blood pressure would get dangerously high every time. I'm trying to compare it to something, anything in my prior life that can compare, and I honestly can't.

I was caught in a cycle of Dialysis. On Monday morning, my dad would convince them not to call an ambulance to send me to the ER, we would pick up a sandwich at Jimmy John's while I puked the entire way home, he'd help me into the house, I'd devour the sandwich (or sometimes two), then I would fall asleep at 4:00 often sleeping until sometime the next afternoon. I would wake up, not knowing what day or time it was, eat something, and fall right back to sleep. Then I would wake up Wednesday and do it all over again.

Looking back on those months, things were so bad, that the second half of my treatments, I often thought that the only reason I would make it till the end, was that I would find a way to commit suicide before I had to come back in two days.

I couldn't tell anyone that though. I was hearing from all my friends and family how lucky I was to be alive. I certainly didn't feel lucky. I had these terrible thoughts brewing in my head and I probably went six weeks not telling anyone. Finally, during one session, Lori, my DaVita social worker came to talk to me (I was in a secluded room because we thought I might do better with the dimmed lights and quiet. Also, probably because I was a distraction to the other patients.) I broke down and told her everything I had been feeling. The nurses went outside to get my dad and we let him know how bad things really were. I felt the worst about that. He had been taking care of me since this all started, and I felt like I was letting him down.

He understood though, he was the one person who had been with me every day and saw what I was going through.

I don't mean for this to start off on such a depressing note, but I think it's important to know where I was to appreciate where I am now. They switched me to a different kind of dialysis. It's called PD, or peritoneal dialysis. I do it seven nights a week, all while I sleep, and it is much easier on my body. I will get into how it works and the maintenance involved later, but I can say I have my life back.

June 3

"What about your other book?"

You're two chapters in and this isn't what you expected. Let's talk about my second book. The one you will probably never get to read.

My first book hadn't even arrived from the printers yet and I was ready to start on a follow-up.

First, it should be known that writing everything down was only the first half, the easy half. Editing and formatting and submitting the cover took forever. Again, thank you to my daughter, Emily, for help with all that. If it wasn't for her, ya'll would've gotten a pile of loose-leaf paper in a Drug Mart bag.

I had plenty more stories to tell. I set some guidelines for myself with the first book: First, the stories had to be about me, if you were disappointed to not see the story about us climbing into old railroad cars and then you falling into the river and ruining your pants, I tried to stick to embarrassing stories about me. There is nothing stopping you from writing your own book (I will be first in line to buy it!) Second, No work stories. Or at least very few. But as I finished it, I realized most of the people I know, I know from relationships that grew from work, either my eighteen years in retail or my four years at Heartland. Those were the stories my friends were asking about, "That time we..." or "That crazy customer..." or "Remember all those bees!"

So, I started working on book number two, *Business Cards: Still (Game)Crazy After All These Years!* It was going to be in the same format as my first one, 52 short stories, each one labeled with a card in the deck.

I ran into a few problems. It was impossible to write about work without talking about old employees and customers. They are the ones who make the work stories interesting. The kid who ran away crying to his mom when I told him, "GameCube says you suck!" or the dozens of teenage employees I fired for theft... Fifty-two chapters is a lot and so no one was safe.

That was another issue, I started with notes to remind me about topics to write about, but when I started, I found that each one wasn't enough to flesh out into multiple pages of worthwhile content. I started combining stories and it worked, but now I didn't have enough to fill up my book.

Another overlying issue, and maybe the most pressing, is that I really thought I was going to die at any time. I started to plan for this. I casually gave out my computer password so people could log in and find my progress and I reached out to co-workers from the past to see if they wanted to contribute chapters about what it was like working together over the years. I thought this would solve the multiple difficulties I was having. They could get their funny memories in. I could fill some pages. And my daughter could collect the stories and finish editing when I was gone.

I should have known this wouldn't go as planned. I learned long ago that whatever your intentions are, the next person will only ever be about fifty percent as invested. I did a lot of fundraising in my time at GameStop and GameCrazy. I came up with, I felt, really good ideas and developed really cool raffles. But no matter how excited I was about them, if I had to rely on others to get behind it, the ideas never caught on. That's how this was going. I reached out to old co-workers, planting the seeds, hoping they would provide short stories about what they remembered fondly, or not so much, from our time together in retail.

I got back a handful of responses, mostly saying they have been trying to forget those years of their lives or reminding me to write "about that one time..." or "that one customer..."

I suppose I didn't explain the assignment well enough, but a text out of the blue, ten years after our last shift together saying, "I'm writing half of a book, but I expect to die before I'm finished. Do you mind finishing it up for me?" would have been kind of confusing.

I was making good progress and had finished about thirteen stories, or one suit, a quarter done. That's when I was sitting at work on the publisher's website and decided I didn't want to publish both a soft-cover book and an e-book version. I clicked on the E-book option and clicked delete. Some sort of warning "Are you sure!?" popped up and I quickly confirmed, "Yeah, idiot. I know what I'm doing!? And both files disappeared. I was devastated that all that work had gone to waste. (Don't ask, the answer is No, I didn't have it backed up anywhere!)

I stewed over my mistake for a few days and complained

to those closest to the project. Everyone assured me that I would be able to rewrite those chapters and they would come out better than before.

Then something even worse happened. By about the third or fourth day, I didn't care anymore...

Looking back, I wasn't really that happy with my work anyway. It wasn't what I wanted to write, it wasn't what I thought people wanted to read, and the only good stories were only entertaining because they were mean spirited about customers or co-workers.

My dad has put it well since I started complaining about work, probably about my very first job as a paperboy, "Work sucks." he would say and change the subject.

Almost a year has gone by. I'm finally able to start writing again. About something that I hope you care about. At least I haven't found much information about kidney disease or dialysis available on the internet. I'm hoping you learn more in the pages of this book than you ever wanted or need to know. I truly hope you or your loved ones never have to deal with this terrible disease.

June 4

After a six-month battle over my insurance coverage, I finally had my initial evaluation for a kidney transplant. This was a pretty important step. Survival rates go up substantially after a transplant, not to mention quality of life. Not having to do dialysis every night would be wonderful.

I had to go to Cleveland Clinic's main campus for this, which meant I called one of my best friends (and currently not working on weekdays) Chris. He was a life saver when I went in for my PD catheter surgery and he came through for me this time as well. I tried to drive myself once in between these visits and got terribly turned around trying to find parking. Every road seems to be one way, and I was always going the wrong way, and any wrong turn took me immediately into the heart of the ghetto. I was fifty minutes late for my appointment. They saw that I was having an anxiety attack, so they took me anyway, but then I missed another appointment I had across town.

Chris, and the nice helpers in the maroon vests, got me where I needed to be and he provided much needed support by sitting in the waiting room, reading his book, and drinking his multiple coffees.

First, I met Amy. She is my transplant coordinator; she was really sweet and explained what I could expect over the next four hours.

Then, someone brought a tablet into the room and sat it on the desk. This was Paula, she was a doctor who would ask me every medical question imaginable to determine if I am strong enough to accept a kidney.

One question that caught me off guard was: "Do you ever think about hurting yourself or wish you were dead?" now, I already mentioned that I broke down to my social worker and my dad that I was really depressed during in center hemodialysis, and they had passed that note on to my primary doctor, so I knew it was in my records somewhere. I told her honestly that I did before but that I was doing much better now. It did make me nervous though, I felt like I was interviewing for my life. These doctors would be having a discussion about who would get on the list based on these answers and I didn't want to hurt my chances.

Another question that was hard to answer was "Who would be taking care of me after the surgery?" I quickly replied, "My wife." After all, I'm looking forward to leaving my parents' and going back home once I don't have to do dialysis anymore. She wanted my wife to call and confirm this plan and so I ended up holding my cell phone up to the tablet so they could talk, neither of them in the room physically. She asked Jeanette if she would be able to stay home from work for six weeks... Oh man, we were not prepared for that at all. Plus, I can't drive after surgery, and I would have to be driven to the main campus, twice a week for the following four weeks. I panicked and hung up on Jeanette and changed my answer to my dad. It looked like I would be at my parents' house for another few months when this was done.

"And what about your backup?"

Jesus, this lady was pushing it. How many unemployed people do you think I know!? I told her my daughter, Ellie, and gave her the phone number. She wouldn't be able to get out of work either, but we would figure it out. I talked with Ellie when I got home that night and told her, in the words of Winston Zeddemore in Ghostbusters, "You say yes!"

We discussed the increased dangers of other health issues associated from being a transplant recipient. The medications I will have to take so that my body doesn't reject the foreign kidney will also diminish my immune system. Cancer, open sores and other pleasant side effects are common.

One of their main concerns was that I have pretty bad GI issues already, GI issues is a polite way of saying that I puke every morning and get terrible diarrhea. These medications will add to those problems for sure. Yet another thing to look forward to.

Then came another bombshell. Once I got a transplant, The Kidney Foundation would no longer be footing the bill to keep my insurance going. If you ever left a job and had to get Cobra, you know it's like eight hundred dollars a month. "How are you going to pay for that?"

"Handies out behind the dumpster!" was probably not what she wanted to hear.

"Um, my dad will help. And I have an aunt..." I trailed off sheepishly.

The rest of the day was pretty straightforward. I went to

the basement for a CT scan and the lab for, what looked like, two hundred vials of blood.

When we were finally done, it was past five o'clock and I was exhausted, ready to go home. This was when Chris came to the rescue again "Do you want to get food before we leave?" He knew I hadn't eaten before we went in, and we never did get a break to get lunch. We went to the mostly empty cafeteria, and each got two pieces of pizza. It wasn't particularly good, but after such a long stressful day, it might have been the best slices I ever had.

And now, I wait.

June 5

This is the obligatory chapter about pee.

After my emergency surgery to insert a catheter in my chest for dialysis, they wheeled me back to the ER. The nurse informed me that I was going to be admitted and that she was going to have to give me a catheter...

"What kind of a wishy-washy place was this? I just came back from getting my catheter. I thought and was about to say, when she lifted up my hospital gown and shoved all eighteen inches of a lubed up (thankfully!) catheter straight into my pee hole.

I have never experienced anything like that before. It hurt and it was surprising. In all his infinite wisdom, Mr. Horse on Ren and Stimpy put it best... "No sir, I don't like it."

When you are bed ridden for two full weeks, hooked up to oxygen and all sorts of other wires and tubes, it is very convenient to have a catheter. Gravity does its job and your urine just kind of drains out into a bag on the side of the bed. You don't have to try, and you don't even really feel it. The nurses come around and see that the bag is full, they measure the quantity (as with everything in such a controlled setting) and they empty it into the toilet.

On about the tenth day of my visit, I was starting to feel better and was about ready to leave. The nurse, came into the room, distracted me with conversation, and yanked the catheter out. It hurt just as much coming out as it did going in, but I had been through hell and was used to it by now.

"Okay, let us know when you have the urge to pee and we'll help you to the bathroom,"

She left me there with my first responsibility in over a week. For so many days, I was living in a constant blur, never really getting any good sleep, just kind of flipping through the channels, eating the bland hospital food they brought me, rolling over when they needed to change the bedding out from underneath me, and peeing into a bag without ever thinking about it. Now, I had two jobs. Drink as much as I could and pee it all out.

And so I drank... And drank... And drank!

But when it was time to pee, nothing happened. I didn't have the urge and nothing came out, despite my greatest efforts.

They came in with a cold jelly (why does it always have to be so cold!?) and an ultrasound machine. They were able to see into my bladder and it was full. It should have been Niagara Falls in there!

And so, as I was discussing our options and what steps we were going to take to keep me from exploding, Big Trouble In Little China style. The nurse grabbed my wiener and shoved another catheter in.. This one was temporary, just to get things moving again. And it worked as advertised. I filled the bag up and she ripped it out again. "We'll try again tomorrow." and she disappeared out of the room.

After a few more days of this, it was clear things were not flowing smoothly. They put a new semi-permanent catheter in, velcroed a bag to my leg, and sent me home.

I was told to measure and empty the contents of the bag a few times a day and we would follow up in four weeks.

One of my many doctor's appointments was with a urology specialist, I arrived a half hour early, thanks to my new full time Uber driver, my dad. I went in, as he stayed in the car, COVID was pretty prevalent at this time. Of course, they couldn't find me in the system. This was the first time I had really been out of the house in a while. I was in pain and getting agitated. I was not leaving without being seen! They figured it out and I went back into a small room to change into a gown. I found, to my horror, why I was in so much pain. The urine bag had loosened its grip and slid down my leg to my calf, stretching the tube to its limit and putting all the weight and pressure onto the tip of my penis.

I was frantically trying to fix this problem when the doctor came in and solved it for me. He nonchalantly ripped it out and tossed the entire thing into the trash.

"Okay, go drink as much as you can and pee every hour for the next six hours and then come back and see me later today."

I let myself out and we went to lunch. I downed three waters and went to the bathroom...

... And nothing.

So we went for a walk to try and stir things up, and I went into the nature center bathroom...

... And nothing.

This happened again at a random McDonald's and again at the doctor office.

My second appointment that day had come. I was back in the same small room, changing into a fresh gown. The doctor came in again. "Okay, all set? Any questions?"

"Um, yeah. I drank a ton of water, like you said. Nothing came out."

"Great, you're free to go. Wait, what!?"

In came a nurse with the jelly and the bladder ultrasound machine. "Yep, you aren't kidding. you're messed up!"

I really didn't want another catheter, I was starting to look like a chopped steak down there. I asked him what my options were.

"Sure, we can put another catheter in or you can leave the urine in there and you'll die." He laid out the choices and gave me time to think it over.

When he returned, he did have one more option. I could use the single-use catheters (like the ones they used in the hospital during those last few days.)

He asked if I would be comfortable inserting that by myself. It was about eighteen inches long. I looked at it in disbelief and confusion and said I didn't know.

We went into the bathroom and washed our hands really good. He pulled me out from under my gown and held me firmly in his hand. "Well, go ahead. slide it in there."

It was pre-lubed, but it was so long. I slid it in a little ways.

"No man. You really got to get it in there!"

"What do you mean? It's in there!"

"You'll know when its far enough."

I pushed farther, it was like a magic trick. My penis (spoiler to the ladies, it is not eighteen inches.) took almost the entire thing. Then it happened. It felt like we reached in and pressed a button (my prostate, maybe?) and the pee came flooding out. "Hey, how neat is that!?"

He quickly left the room and fetched me a gift. because I did so well, he gave me a sealed box full of these catheters.

"Use these every four hours and keep trying to urinate on your own every hour or so. Come back and see me in two weeks."

I cleaned up, changed back into my pants, and went to the receptionist. I was tired, ready to go home.

"Cal!?" It was my friend, Jim's girlfriend, Lori. I didn't recognize her with her mask on and didn't expect to see anyone I knew in this environment.

"Oh, hey Lori." I said. slightly embarrassed with a huge box of catheters under my arm.

"Hey, what are you doing here!? How are you!?"

"I'm great. I'm certainly not here because my wiener is broken and will probably never work right again. I had such a great time here today. Let's schedule another date in a few weeks." Lori is wonderful and sweet as can be. But in that office, on that day, I was not in the mood to catch up.

The following weeks were pretty hard on me. I didn't like using the catheters, so I would only do it when I felt like I was full. Which usually would happen at three in the morning. I would wake up, feeling extra bloated and run to the bath-room in a panic, thinking that tonight would be the night my bladder ruptured and my body filled with urine, poisoning me from the inside.

After a few weeks, things started to flow again. One after-noon I came screaming out of the bathroom. My dad jumped out of his chair thinking something was wrong.

"We did it! We did it!" I yelled and waved my arms in my best Woody impression from the end of Toy Story.

I called the next day and canceled my follow up with the urology doctor. My co-pays were piling up and the hour drive up to Cleveland was tough on both me and my dad. I've been peeing like a champ ever since. I'll take all the small victories I can get.

June 6

After two weeks in the hospital, they were getting tired of me, and I was stable and ready to go home. Well, not home exactly, just ready to get out of there.

I don't remember asking and the conversation might have gone on behind my back. I was going to stay with my parents for a while to give me time to heal and build up my strength. One of the reasons was that I was too weak to drive, and I was starting in-center dialysis three days a week. There is a DaVita center in Wooster, about ten minutes from my parents' house. My dad is retired and would be able to drop me off and, more importantly, pick me up after.

Dad set up a bed in the dining room for me because I wasn't strong enough to get upstairs to the bedroom which had always been his PlayStation 3, NCAA Football, weight-lifting room. My stuff, although I didn't have much, filled the table and that entire side of the main floor. He brought an old recliner in from the garage and squeezed it in between each of theirs.

And I slept. And ate big bowls of chili occasionally, it was a cold winter and I had to eat tons of protein to help my bed sore heal faster. And then I slept some more. I was completely wiped out from my hospital stay and also from my continued dialysis every other day.

It turned out the rides my dad would provide were much more important than I originally thought. When I finished my sessions, they were 10:00 to 3:00, I was a mess. The nurses often gathered around me after I was unhooked and stood up, I would pass out and fall back into my seat. They would run out into the snow to get my dad from the car and try to call an ambulance to take me to the emergency room. Dad would convince them not to and explain that I usually felt better after I puked the whole way home, ate a sandwich, and slept the next twenty hours. They would reluctantly agree and he helped me slink out to the car with my walker. I will never be able to properly explain how bad those dialysis days were. No one, besides my dad will ever truly understand what I was going through! He starts every conversation about anything medical with "I don't know nothing but..." And even he knew these treatments were killing me.

As terrible as my new existence was, it was made worse by the fact that I was an hour from my wife, kids, and friends. My parents are delightful, but I needed more at that time. A few friends came down to see me, but I don't think anyone understood just how bad things really were. I've never been the type of person to put myself out there and ask for help.

It was great to find that an old friend from GameStop had also recently moved to Wooster for work.

Vince saw a random post on Facebook and reached out. What started as a "Yeah, we'll make it happen sometime..." quickly turned into, "Please Vinnie, save me from this house!" (That's my dad's joke, not mine.)

He picked me up after work and we went out to Longhorn. It was definitely one of those dinners where neither of us ate very much of our steak and spent over two hours catching up on lost time. It had been about ten years and we had so much to go over.

We have since become movie buddies, going to see Jackass Forever (but not on opening night, because of a snowstorm that closed down the entire town), The Batman (He insisted we drive an hour for that one, we went to the IMAX on opening night, instead of The Diaper, as he calls our local theater), and not Morbius (No matter how many times they try to release it in theaters!)

After five months, I got surgery to put a PD catheter in my stomach and I did the two weeks of training to start doing my dialysis at home. One of the aspects of that is keeping everything sterile. Which means no pets in the room at night and I was supposed to be set up in a closed room, meaning not the dining room. My mom was delighted when we cleaned all the crap out of that room, moving half out to bins in the garage and half upstairs to my dad's game room.

It was nice to have a little bit of privacy and it was getting warmer so he didn't mind moving his game out to the garage, it's more like a mancave.

We were waiting for "the shipment" of PD supplies and my dad cleaned out two drawers of his dresser in my new room. We were all set, waiting for the delivery so I could start my nightly routine...

Vince, I know you give me lots of credit for hiring you when you first came to Cleveland from New York, but I'm so glad I did. Thank you for being a good friend.

June 7

...With two empty dresser drawers, we were ready to accept our initial shipment of PD dialysis supplies. They had asked us if we had room set aside and we did have an almost empty closet. We'd be fine, I assured the nurses.

We waited all afternoon and the delivery never showed up. I called and they informed me that the driver called off sick. That was Tuesday, they rescheduled it for Thursday.

Thursday arrived and so did a full-size moving truck! The delivery man had three pallets, two thousand pounds of supplies for me. We certainly were not prepared for this much. We didn't have the room and Dad was convinced the house couldn't structurally hold that much wait on the second floor. In a panic, we directed him into the basement. He had a cool, robotic dolly that was able to go down the stairs with ease. This impressed me greatly since I consider the ED-209 to be the pinnacle of futuristic technology and even that can't handle steps!

He put that dolly to work, making forty trips down into the cellar. My dad frantically shifted stuff around and piled the boxes neatly against the wall. Not knowing what I'll need, they order extra of everything. There are two ways to do PD dialysis, manual and with the cycler. Manual uses gravity to fill my stomach cavity with fluid and then drains it out, the cycler machine, which I would mostly be using, uses suction to fill and drain and keeps track of all the math for me so I don't need scales to weigh and tell me how effective my sessions are. Even though I wouldn't ever use those supplies, they had to send out the manual equipment in case of a power outage or other emergency.

I held the door.

After that shipment, I called Sherry, my PD nurse, and she visited the house to make sure I was all set. She also brought the cycler machine along with a stand. I'm told this machine is ten grand which meant two things. First, I had to sign a contract saying that it was on loan to me and if I got a transplant, I wasn't allowed to sell it on Ebay. Second, Dad didn't want anything to do with it. Sherry asked him to carry it upstairs and he refused. "If anyone is going to drop that thing down the stairs, it's not going to be me!"

This machine isn't light, and this wasn't the first time Sherry had to carry one up a flight of stairs.

She put the stand together with ease and inspected my room with a checklist of questions about the house. She wanted to make sure I was prepared for what I was getting myself into. It's a little too late for doubts, I did have a tube poking out of a hole in my stomach, after all.

Dad carried heavy boxes of fluid up from the basement to stock my closet with a few days' worth of solution. Each box has two bags of six thousand milliliters of fluid, Yellow has 1.5% dextrose (essentially sugar), Green has 2.5% and Red has 4.25%. I use one bag of yellow and one green every night. I'm fortunate that I don't get bad swelling. When you do, that's when you would use the red bag. The more dextrose, the more toxins it pulls out of your system when it drains. Also, the harder it is on your body and the worse you feel the next morning. They say, "kidney disease gives you the hangover but without the drinking."

She was happy with what she saw. My training was done. I was never going back to doing hemodialysis again.

I do feel a million times better on PD dialysis and I have my days and energy back. But everything is not rainbows and butterflies. Dad has to carry those boxes up every few days, he works it into his workout schedule. I have to carry the bags of fluid into the bathroom every morning, cut them open and empty my stomach juices into the toilet. Then I have about thirty minutes of set-up every evening before bed.

Anytime I feel overwhelmed with the amount of upkeep, I remind myself that the alternative is much worse.

If I don't do it every night, I literally die...

Or worse yet, end up back on hemodialysis.

June 8

"When there's no one left in the living world
who remembers you,
you disappear from this world.
We call it the Final Death."

-Coco (Disney/Pixar, 2017)

I met Chad Brickley all the way back at Babbage's. That was GameStop before they bought Software Etc, Funcoland, and others and changed the names. I started working there in September of '99 for the Dreamcast launch. This must have been around then.

He would come in with his friends and buy everything, and I mean everything. But that's not what I remember about our earliest interactions. It was how he paid for all his games. He kept crumpled up dollar bills in all of his pockets. They were never-ending, like a magician's handkerchief, He would empty pocket after pocket onto the counter and we would count them up and flatten them out together.

Some of his friends called him Alan. I'm not sure why. I think that was his first name and Chad was his middle, but I can't say for certain. He also went by Hoth Beast. that is the snow monster at the beginning of Empire Strikes back. I'm not sure where that came from either, but he embraced it, making it his e-mail address.

Chad was very generous. He worked as a tech at Dave & Buster's. One of his responsibilities was to clean out the coin push games after the busy weekends. He would empty those machines and end up with pockets full of coins at the end of his shift. He knew my wife and I liked going there on dates and so he would bring me gallon size Ziplock bags full of coins. We had to sneak the coins in because their currency was card based, each swipe got you seven coins. We had thousands. We were able to play for hours, cleaning out the tickets from multiple machines. Then we cashed in the tickets for X-Box games, which I would exchange to my store for games that Chad wanted for an extreme discount, which I then used for lunch, it was the circle of life.

One time he gave us "Free Dinner" cards for the Dave & Buster's restaurant. We took them in and enjoyed our meals. When the check came, I handed the waitress the two cards and she looked at them, confused. She left us to get the manager.

"Where did you get those cards?" he asked.

I knew something was wrong, so I thought quick, "Oh, I won those in a poker game."

"Those are incentives we give out to the employees when they do a good job. They aren't for customers. We're actually missing a stack and I'd like to know who took them."

"Sorry, I just pulled them from a pot with a pair of pocket Jacks."

"Alright." He said, looking my wife and I over with disapproval. "But you have to pay for your food."

That was a bummer. We ordered the most expensive dinners on the menu since we thought they were free.

Chad worked for me at GameCrazy. I had just started managing the store and wanted his business as much as I needed an employee. He got our discount and free movie and game rentals at Hollywood Video, and I was sure he would buy all his games from me. A perfect plan!

I'll say it was fun working with him. We had demos set up throughout the store and we played Mario Kart: Double Dash for hours. A Hollywood customer actually called the corporate complaint line because we were so loud one night. We beat Metal Slug 3, a super hard game for the old X-Box without continues. Kevin, our DM at the time, was so proud of us!

One of the cool benefits of working for Hollywood Video was that the DVD's came in six days before release, on Wednesday for the following Tuesday. We were allowed to take them home and watch them early so that we could recommend them to customers at release. Or, in Chad's case, he took them all home and burned copies for himself and his friends. The problem was that he didn't work very often and always returned them late. This was a point of contention between me and Bill, the Hollywood manager. He was trying to keep his stock ready on release days and I was trying to keep my staff under control.

I'll never forget, it was Lost Boys 2 (Yes, there is a sequel and yes, it sucks). They would get like twenty copies of a lot of movies, so it didn't really matter if one was missing on Tuesday morning, it was annoying, but the customers didn't know the difference. But we only had one copy of that particular movie. Of course, someone was waiting for us to open that morning to rent it, but it wasn't there. Bill came over and complained that he got chewed out by the customer and I called Chad in a fury of rage. "Get that movie back here. Right now!'

He was upset that he had to drive five miles to the store on his day off to return it, but he must have known, by the tone of my voice, that I was serious.

When he arrived, I told him that his rental privileges were revoked for a month. I had to let both him and, more importantly, Bill know that I meant business. Returning the early movies on time was a rule but there wasn't really a defined punishment in place for when it happened. It was kind of just accepted. Chad questioned the severity of the punishment immediately. "Really, you're taking my rentals away!?"

"Yes. And you're lucky that's all I'm taking away." I had to stand firm.

"I quit." He said and walked back out to his car. This might have been the original mic drop.

Surprisingly we didn't stay angry at each other for long. GameCrazy went out of business with Hollywood Video and I returned to GameStop. And I was back in Chad's neighborhood. He was back to buying everything and I was lenient on him when he had to return games, either because they were no good or because he had over spent that month and needed money for groceries.

Sometimes, when it was really hot, he wouldn't leave his house and I would deliver his games to him. The other side of that coin was that we both read The Walking Dead comic as the individual issues came out and he would let me borrow it each month.

Some of the best memories I had with Chad were our many Super Mario World Tournaments throughout the years. It was one of our favorite games and so, naturally, we found ways to compete to see who the best player was. First, we raced to see who could beat all 96 levels the fastest, this was decades before "speed-running" was a thing. After finding it difficult to get so many televisions and Super Nintendo's together in one place, we took turns playing levels, eliminating players whenever they lost a life in the game. These were great nights of gaming that went on for hours. Chad was always very nice. He would have loved to play other games but knew I was only any good at Mario and tolerated playing the same game all the time.

The last time I heard from Chad was on a Friday night when I lived in my apartment building. We had a movie theater room on the first floor and Friday was movie night. He called and asked if we were watching anything, but I was driving back from a work trip to Michigan.

That was August of 2019. He passed away that weekend.

I never did get the full details of what happened and I missed the funeral because I was sick.

I called his roommate to ask if there was anything I could do to help him or Chad's family. He had me call the comic shop to let them know.

I told them the news and they were understandably upset. He was as good of a customer and friend there as he was with me. He liked comics and games equally. I told them to check his file and return the books to the sales floor. I was devastated to learn that the only comic he was still requesting was The Walking Dead each month. The one he shared with me...

Everyone knows hindsight is 20/20 but we should have seen this as a sign.

I don't claim to know much. If you've read both books, there are over eighty stories to prove that.

One thing I do know is that I miss Chad dearly.

He loved his friends and he was kind and generous to everyone he knew.

I will never forget him.

June 9

"We want to throw you a fundraiser." It was my friend Kate. She called me the week prior with her idea. I had worked with her at GameStop, and her sister, Jess, at Heartland, and their cousin, Jason, at GameCrazy. They've always been good friends, but this was unexpected.

I wasn't sure how to respond. I'm not the type who has an easy time asking for help. Much of my PD training involved my nurse convincing me to call the on-call nurse or the number on the machine if I had any trouble during the night. "I'm sure it'll be okay to wait until morning, I don't want to bother anybody." "Godamn, Godamn! Call them! It's their job to help you. And if you don't, it'll probably get infected, and you'll end up in the hospital."

I agreed to put my pride behind my finances, which were a mess, as you can imagine. I had to stop working when this all started in November. I applied for disability, which takes six months to kick in. (And an extra month, because it goes by complete calendar months, and my last day at work was November 2.) They hadn't worked out the details yet, they didn't want to plan everything and have me say I wasn't interested. We met for dinner at a restaurant/bar run by their family. (Shout out to TEAMZ in Middleburg Heights, Ohio. The best damn wings in the world, according to my son.)

It was honestly great to see them. I had seen Kate and Jess often, but it had been years since I talked with Jason. It was one of those times where the waitress had to remind us to order, or we would have sat there all night without ever glancing at our menus.

They had already done most of the leg work. Jason knew how much each person's meal and drink tickets would cost and how much we would charge. He also picked the perfect day and time. Friday, August 12, the first pre-season game of the year for the Browns. We'd have the party room for us and be able to reach out to the bar as well. Kate and Jess knew how to create an event on Facebook, and we discussed raffle basket ideas, 50/50 raffles and sideboards. My only contribution was that we should have a squares board for the football game. My family loves squares and we've missed playing it the last few Superbowl parties.

I have high hopes that this will be successful. I do know that it'll be a great time and I look forward to getting together with friends and family.

I tried to express my gratitude, but I doubt they could ever truly understand how much this means to me. A common problem with this disease is that very few people understand what dialysis is and what we go through. It is a very lonely disease. My virtual support groups through the DaVita app help, but it's different coming from people who I know.

Tonight, I felt loved.

June 10

If Grover was here, he would tell you to skip this chapter.

I have to talk about health insurance for a moment... I know, I know! But it's important and if you ever get really sick, you might need to know what I went through, what I'm still going through, seven months later.

I had only been at my new job for three months when this all started. That was part of the problem, my insurance didn't kick in until November and so I was waiting to see a doctor. Everyone yelled at me for waiting so long. But really think about it. People don't go to the doctor without insurance, no matter how hurt or sick, or in my case, swollen they are.

My boss was really concerned. She was texting me often while I was in the hospital. I was a manager for twenty years. I knew that she also needed to know when and if I was coming back to work. I pushed back this conversation as long as I could with short, dismissive text responses. Finally, well into the second week, I had to call her and tell her I wasn't going to come back. She felt bad for my situation, and I felt bad for leaving them in a lurch. I was just getting the hang of the job and it was a very small payroll department, the others would have to pick up the slack and they would have to hire and train another person. I was very emotional during that hospital stay and I broke down to my boss over the phone. It was awkward, but I'm sure she understood. We were never very close to begin with and we haven't talked since that day. I'm curious how they handled it, but not enough to stop up and check on them.

When you stop working, you obviously lose the benefits. This wasn't good since I provided the insurance for the family, and I needed it now more than ever. If you've ever looked over the Cobra paperwork when you left a job, they offer to continue your medical coverage at your own expense. You have to pay your half as well as the half that the company was traditionally paying. It can be hundreds, or close to a thousand dollars a month. Did they not get the memo that I need Cobra because I am newly unemployed?

I feel like I'm thanking a lot of people throughout these chapters, and I've probably mentioned them already, but DaVita has saved my life in so many ways. My social worker explained that The Kidney Foundation would foot the bill for my insurance. She had me sign the right forms in the right places and she took care of the rest. There were two possible scenarios for how this was going to work. Either they were going to send in the check each month or I was going to pay it and they would reimburse me the amount. Thankfully, I was never asked, and they did it the first way. I didn't really have the money to send in and wait for the check to come back to me.

It was supposed to take four to six weeks for the insurance to start and so it wasn't alarming when the receptionists at the doctors' offices told me my insurance claims were denied and I would have to pay out of pocket. "No, I'm good. It'll go through next month we just have to resubmit." I was getting used to explaining.

As time went on, I started to get nervous, but my social worker assured me that it just took time. Finally, the DaVita insurance counselor, Joanna, got involved. She worked out of West Virginia, so we worked exclusively over the phone. We called the insurance company together to find out what was taking so long. After much confusion, it was established that they received the checks from the National Kidney Foundation... And threw them away! They then claimed that since I didn't sign up fast enough, it was too late, and I was out of luck.

Yeah, Joanna wasn't going to accept that answer. She had copies of everything we sent in with timestamps. (Keep your receipts, kids!) She had the checks reprinted and got everything worked out. I know she fought so hard for me because she cares about me, but it also helps that I owe Davita tens of thousands of dollars and the only way they were going to see any of that was if this got resolved.

The bills never stopped piling up and everyone was so happy to hear from me when I finally had my insurance card. I called them all and had them resubmit the claims, and there were a lot of claims. I then started getting adjusted bills with actual out-of-pocket amounts, but many of these were already sent to collections by mistake. It was hard to remember which ones I had paid and settled, which ones I had put on a payment plan, and which ones I was "letting ride".

One in particular that was extremely frustrating was for

supplies that a nurse ordered for my bed sore. I wasn't able to apply the bandages by myself and she stopped coming out to the house when my insurance was first denied. All this crap was sitting, unopened in the garage and a collection agency was calling three times a week for a hundred and fifteen dollars. This was a small enough amount that I was going to pay it with my debit card to get them to stop calling. When I reached for my wallet, however, I realized I had left it out in the car.

"Do you want to run and get it?" The woman asked, "I'd like to close your case for our client."

"Yeah, I'm not really running anywhere these days. Let me call you back."

Later that afternoon, wallet in hand, I returned the call. I had some time to think things through though and I asked for the medical company's name and phone number. I called them and fought through the options for a while. "Dispute a claim!" I yelled into my speaker phone. When I finally got a human on the other end, I explained my situation.

"Oh, yes. It says right here we submitted it to your insurance last month and we're waiting to send you a reduced bill."

"Well, I'm glad I didn't pay the debt collector that's been harassing me almost every day!"

"Oh yeah. That's a mistake. You shouldn't pay them. I'll note the account. Thank you for calling. Please hold for the survey."

You bet your ass I held for the survey! I want to know how many people just pay these people to get them to stop. Also, how difficult it is to call for a refund when that happens. How will they feel when I call them every day!?

It's all just very stressful.

June 11

It's interesting how peoples' interests and passions can change. Less than a year ago, I was obsessed with the possibility of Kill Bill 3 and the highlight of my week was Pizza Tuesdays at the office. Today I was very busy, but my entire day revolved around dialysis patients.

My morning started like most mornings do. I wake up with the sun, at about seven, but I can't get out of bed yet, because I have to be on the machine for eleven hours. I stayed up late last night and so I was stuck in my room until about nine thirty. The dialysis machine was chirping away loudly, making it difficult to fall back asleep, so I hopped on Facebook. Most of my feed is posts from kidney disease support groups, while it used to be predominantly Sega Genesis and horror movie fan clubs.

A woman asked for advice about choosing hemo (in-center) or PD dialysis. She was meeting with her doctors and wanted to know what to expect and what questions to ask. I messaged her with my phone number and offered to explain the pros and cons of each. She messaged back asking if I was also in London! I told her that I was in Cleveland, Ohio, and specified that is in the US. We continued messaging throughout the day. She asked how bad the surgery was, how uncomfortable the fluid is when it dwells in my stomach, Am I still able to do the things I did before and am I able to go "on holiday." I answered her honestly, Surgery was fine. You don't really notice it. I do on PD but not on hemo. And I have never gone "on holiday." She is going to update me on her decision after she talks with the doctor.

I had some testing at my dialysis center. I only go in twice a month now and I actually look forward to seeing Sherry, my PD nurse, and the nurses that I used to give so much trouble when I was spending fifteen hours a week in that awful chair. They are truly happy to see that I'm doing so well, and also that they don't have to deal with me passing out on them all the time. My eyes would often roll back into my head, and I would throw up into my mask, it was gross.

Today, they had me talk with a woman who was unsure about making the jump to PD. I sat with her and explained my situation. It was a little different for me because my body was not handling my in-center sessions well at all. I would have done literally anything to get out of going there anymore. She was handling it okay, except that she was so exhausted afterwards that she slept her days away and never had time for anything. I understood her hesitance, there really isn't much information available on the subject and the doctors can explain it the best they know how, but it's different hearing it from someone who has been living it. I invited her and her husband over to see me set up the machine for the night and see all the storage required in the basement. We realized we live right around the block from each other. Whichever decision she makes, I hope I was able to answer her questions.

After my afternoon with Sherry, I got out just in time to jump on a virtual support group. We have a pretty tight group at this point, about four of us are regulars, and a few patients have been joining for the first time. I'm on so many of them that the moderator asked if I had any feedback for her to take back to the person in charge of the project. The only advice I had was that they need to advertise it better. Those of us who use it, really get a lot out of it, but not nearly enough people know about it. These support groups have a set of rules, which are all pretty standard. Share the floor, keep it confidential, participate, don't multitask, and one that I think about a lot...

Use "I" statements. The example they use is "Blue is my favorite color." instead of "Blue is the best color!"

Sure, I might think blue is the best color, but I shouldn't be making people feel bad about their opinions. Just like *I* think hemodialysis is miserable and worse than death, but I have to respect the opinions of others and not make them feel bad about their choices. Even if they are clearly wrong,

Some things are simply fact and should be above dispute. Maybe they like the color yellow best. Yeah, yellow sucks.

Or maybe they like Terminator 2 more than the first one. You know, the one where the Terminator has to baby-sit and isn't allowed to kill anyone. Terminator will always be superior to the tame sequel!

All hate mail can be sent to Crazycal179@sbcglobal.net. I'll know which guys read this far.

June 12

It's 3:20 in the morning. I woke up two hours ago, at 1:30 to my dialysis machine screaming at me with a "Low Pressure!" warning. It was making a new hissing sound from the back. I hit "Try again" and the green timer started ticking down. The same warning appeared, "Low Pressure!" I switched out the bag on top of the machine and tried again. This time it said "M71.1 pneumatic Alarm!" Disconnect and call the number on the machine. I did as I was told and worked through the prompts. No, I don't want to order supplies!

"Hello, thank you for calling. Can I get your name, please?" Her name was Manny, my cousin's name. I wondered if it's spelled the same. It's late and we were both tired, I didn't ask. After going over a few possible quick fixes, none of them worked, she wanted me to power down the machine and start over with all new supplies.

A quick note about life on PD dialysis: My cords don't reach from my room to the bathroom. So, every time I have to go to the bathroom, I have to unhook from the machine, do my business, and run back before the next stage starts. Many nights, I have lost track of time and the machine is ready to empty the fluid from my stomach, the alarm goes off and I have to run down the hall and plug back in. The cycler machine is my all-powerful, all-knowing ruler. I never disobey my master!

Against my better judgement, I had to use the bathroom desperately, I had for a few hours, but it's always like camping in the winter for me now. You know when you are so warm in your sleeping bag, and you'll hold it until morning to avoid leaving your tent and going out into the cold. I knew this was going to take a long time, so I told her I'd have to call her back. I was glad when she answered the next time, so I didn't have to explain myself a second time or read off the serial numbers from the machine again.

We went through the motions of "turning it off and back on again." I've seen IT Crowd, I knew that much, at least! It was giving off a loud hissing noise from the back of the machine which I assured Manny was not normal. The machine has a green countdown clock when it is thinking, and this repeated numerous times before turning red with a new warning. "M01-21" ("PC load letter! What the fuck does that mean!?")

We tried this a few times and I kept mentioning the hissing from the back. She finally gave up and ordered me a new machine to be delivered tomorrow. "Do you have the supplies to do manual?" she asked.

Ugh, I hadn't even thought of that. "No... well yeah. It's all in the basement. I've never even taken it out of the boxes." I answered honestly.

"Are you going to continue your treatment tonight?"

"No. I'll do it tomorrow." I answered, only half honestly this time. I can't carry those boxes up two flights of stairs and I wasn't going to bother my dad at this hour.

She walked me through how to ship the broken machine back in the replacement's box and I thanked her for everything she tried to do to help.

We hung up, and I was alone...

A common thread in my support groups and probably throughout this book is the feeling of loneliness that comes with this disease. It is the worst when I'm unable to sleep, sitting up in bed, scratching because my phosphorous is too high, the sun doesn't seem like it will ever rise.

"The callous on my right foot is getting worse with all this walking I'm doing. I should show that to my physical therapist tomorrow. Or at least get a referral to see a new foot doctor since my old foot doctor was with a different hospital and he's no longer there anyway."

"I have a virtual doctor visit at seven. Thank goodness it's not in person, I could never get up and drive the hour up to Cleveland to see her. I'm going to be a tired mess as it is."

"This is an appointment that we had to reschedule because I got lost trying to find parking the last time I went to the main campus of the hospital. I'm not sure, but that was the closest I've ever come to having a panic attack. Oh man, I have two tests scheduled there later this month. Of course, they couldn't fit them both on the same day."

"I wonder if Chris would mind driving me to either or both of those appointments. No, he's been great lately. It would be wrong to ask. I just have to suck it up and figure it out."

"Is that callous going to prevent me from getting on the transplant list?"

These are just some of the pressing thoughts that are racing through my brain right now. "They mostly come out at night... mostly."

It's 4:30 now. My alarm is set for 6:45 for my zoom appointment. I'm going to get some sleep. But I'm hesitant, because I know I'm just going to lay there. I had a nurse who told me about how her sister had kidney disease... But she died! Her dialysis day fell on a holiday. She missed one session and she died the next day. "But you should be fine as long as you never miss." Yeah, that didn't scare the crap out of me or anything. That's what I'll be thinking about as my dialysis machine sits in the corner, powered down, waiting for the replacement to arrive.

Sweet dreams. Don't let the bed bugs bite.

June 13

\I started working when I was in the third grade. I got a paper route for the weekly newspaper, The Sun Herald, delivering to about sixty houses in my neighborhood. I also started mowing lawns a year or so later. I haven't taken a day off in the thirty-five years since.

I spent thirty years in retail and the last five in an office. (At a big boy job.) I never knew any other way. One time I quit a job with my two-week notice, finishing up on a Friday. But they couldn't find anyone to work the weekend, so I worked Saturday and Sunday. Then I started my new job on Monday.

Ozzy says, "No Rest for the Wicked!"

And I had a boss when I worked at a furniture store who said, "You better be making money every minute you're awake. And when you sleep, you better be dreaming of ways to make money when you wake up." Equally potent, but not quite as catchy of a song title.

It's been very difficult not being able to work these past six months. And when I had to quit my job with The Reserves Network, I felt terrible about not giving them more notice.

I was almost dying in a hospital bed and that's what I was worrying about.

I've just started looking for work again. Just something part time. There are strict rules about how much I can earn before it interferes with disability. Although disability takes six months to start, so I'm not sure what they expect people to do in the meantime.

I was happy to be feeling better enough, and consistently each morning to be able to start searching for a job. But I am still very limited as to what I'm able to do. Some of my criteria for my search was that it couldn't have any heavy lifting, I couldn't work too early in the morning, and I couldn't work too late. Oh, and I can't stand for too long or really walk at all and I don't have Wi-Fi so I can't work remote... But other than that, I'm your man!

I stumbled across an app called Papa. They work with health insurance companies. Older patients can request visits for different types of services. If they need help with light cleaning tasks around the house, or rides to the supermarket, or just companionship they request what they want, and "pals" can search through the app and claim the visits. They did a background check, and I watched a virtual informational video, and I was ready to go.

My first try searching the app showed no results within a hundred miles. I thought maybe it just hadn't made it to my area yet. But then, I checked the next day and there were plenty of options available. The site shows the "papa's" name and age and approximate miles away they are from my current location. They selected what services they were looking for help with from a list. Some of the choices included transportation, pet care, companionship, but most of them selected help around the house. Only after accepting the visit does it give their full name, address, and phone number.

I was hesitant to commit to any because I am disabled and can't even do chores around my own house, let alone a stranger's. I eventually picked a visit that was the next morning. Then I noticed the time, 7;30. That was way too early for me, I usually wasn't off of my dialysis machine until ten. I immediately clicked on "cancel visit."

"Are you sure? Canceling leaves a negative experience for the papa and may affect your ability to take jobs in the future."

Yes, cancel.

I looked again and found a woman with the heart icon, companionship. Followed by the house icon, chores. I didn't know if the order of the icons reflected their priorities. Maybe, they mostly wanted someone to spend time with and help with household chores was an afterthought. I selected this one and was provided with a name, address, and phone number. I called her to confirm our visit, thinking she would be happy for anyone to come out at all, because if I didn't take it, most likely, no one was going to so close to the deadline.

"Hello, my name is Cal. I'd like to make sure you're still available for your Papa visit."

"What can you do!?" She asked immediately.

"Um, I can play Scrabble." I answered, feeling inadequate.

"The last guy was hauling this big pile of mulch into my back woods. He hasn't called me back yet."

"No shit, lady! We're not a landscaping company." I didn't dare say out loud. "You'll probably want to try to request him. Good luck." I said and hung up the phone.

"Are you sure? Canceling leaves a negative experience for the papa and may affect your ability to take jobs in the future." The app asked me for the second time in less than ten minutes.

Yes, cancel. I wasn't off to a very good start.

Finally, I found a woman who needed a ride to the eye doctor. She was nervous to drive after her eye surgery. I picked her up, the doctor was less than five minutes down the road and I waited for her in the waiting room. It was a very nice experience, and I gave her a copy of my book as a parting gift.

Next, I found a job with a fifteen-dollar bonus attached to it. I still don't know why some of them have bonuses, but it might be that they are short notice requests. It was far, but it was a five hour day and it was only for companionship, not yard work. I parked a few houses down the street, waiting for the visit to start at 12:30 and took a moment to review the app one last time before going in.

Recommended activities:

-Play games

-Watch movies

Notice: Dementia

I walked up the front stairs with my cane. I think his wife was nervous when she saw me at the door.

"He's a fall risk and you can't leave him alone."

"I'll stay with him and walk with him if he has to walk

to the bathroom." I'm also a fall risk, so if he goes tumbling down the few stairs to the split level, I'm not going to do much besides cushion his fall when I land underneath him.

We sat for a moment and then I asked him if he wanted to play any games.

"Boy, I'm ninety years old. I haven't played games in eighty years. You want to go out back and play kick the can!?"

I learned at that moment that the app just listed generic advice for everyone and that it wasn't specific to the individual clients. Thanks Papa. You made me look like an idiot in front of my new friends. We sat together and talked while his wife volunteered at a local museum for the afternoon. At one point he walked around the living room as I spotted him and held his oxygen hose up and out of his way. Then he took a short nap after I helped lift his legs into bed.

Overall, we both had a very nice day. I liked hearing his life story as much as he liked having someone to tell it to. I saw his name on the list for two upcoming Tuesdays and I snatched them both up.

I really like this app and the freedom it offers me to take work when I'm available.

I look forward to all the different people I'll get to meet.

June 14

We're two weeks into this month-long project and it's time to talk about the elephant in the room. I don't want to save it for the end, because I don't want it to end on such a downer.

This book can be traced back to that day in early November last year when I thought I was dying. I've been thinking about that over the last few months, but it has been difficult to discuss with the people I love and so I'm going to get it out of the way here and now.

I want to start by saying that I'm not afraid to die. After months of feeling as bad as I did last year, I had come to accept the inevitable. I also want to be very clear when I say that I don't want to die. I think there is a difference between those two thoughts that people don't always understand.

I don't take everyday things for granted like I used to. I celebrate nice, sunny days and I find myself complimenting people whenever I have the chance. I think about the few times in my life that I really could have died and how the world would be different without me.

I was in two major car accidents in my life. One when I was in high school and a really bad one two years ago where my car flipped over.

I often think back to the one in high school. If I would have died, I would have never met my wife, Jeanette, who at the time was ready to move back to Texas. Her life would have been completely different. Better? Who's to say. I know one thing though, my kids would have never been born, and that, I can promise you, would have been a tragedy.

At the time of that accident, I was young and thought I was invincible, as all teenagers do. My friends even joked that I might be a Highlander and I could only die if you cut off my head. "There can be only one!" they yelled down the hallway in school after me.

I don't know if this is resonating with you, as the reader. Try to think back to when you were truly in danger and think of how different things would have been if you wouldn't have survived. I hope you are realizing that things would have been worse for the people who love you.

The second, and much more serious, crash left me with a broken rib and pelvic bone. I was rushed to the hospital and spent the night there. I think they let me go home too early and I was in terrible pain. Everyone rushed to tell me how lucky I was to be alive. I didn't feel lucky. When I looked back on that day, I had the feeling that I had done everything I was going to do in life, and it wouldn't have made a difference if that would have been the end.

Sure, my family and friends would have been sad. But time heals all wounds. People would have forgotten about me and moved on. I would have lived forty good years, given the world three amazing kids, and kidney disease would have never crossed my mind.

Being that last November was the third time, that I

can recall, (I'm sure my close friends can remind me of other times, mostly involving lighter fluid at cookouts in the Metroparks.) where I'm surprised to have made it, it's time to discuss how I would like it handled when the time actually does arrive. Of course, I'll be gone, so I guess it doesn't matter what I want...

I don't want anything fancy, and I don't want anything in a church. If you know me, you know I'm not religious at all. Whatever there is, people should feel awkward and over-dressed if they show up in a tie, unless it's laundry day and you don't have any other clean clothes. If the weather is nice, maybe a cookout and kickball game. Or, if it's raining, get together and watch a movie.

I am claustrophobic, even though "I've never even looked at another guy!" (You should watch Turtles from 1990.) so I really don't want to be buried. Cremated and spread at places I used to like.

I don't really have much stuff and nothing of value, any of my nerdy friends can take that crap, or sell it for quarters at a garage sale. But don't let it sit in boxes in the basement collecting dust. If someone can get enjoyment out of it, I want them to.

Finally, if it's not too much trouble or expense, I like those memorial benches in the valley. But it has to say something clever and not "Generously donated by..." It should be something personal to me, like "Everything's coming up Milhouse!" or "Pizza Dude's got thirty seconds." or even "Godamn, Go-damn!"

Sorry if this one made you feel uncomfortable. I'm trying to be honest and write what I'm thinking about and having the doctors call it End Stage Kidney Failure kind of makes me think about it.

Oh, and I'd like any future revenue from this and my first book to be evenly divided between my daughter, Emily, and Kenny, my cover artist. I appreciate both of their help and there literally wouldn't be a book without them. It won't be much so don't get crazy and be dicks about it. And if it does get too complicated just donate it to The Kidney Foundation.

The next three chapters are going to be for my children. If you want to complain about that, I invite you to write your own book and you can write about whatever you want. But I also did the math and if this book comes out at fifteen dollars, as expected, and there are thirty days in June, each entry costs fifty cents. Skip the next three chapters, jump to June 18, and send me an email. I will ask you a question from one of these chapters to confirm you didn't read them. If you get the question wrong, I will send you a buck fifty. Or you can cash that credit in towards two free Butts Up! shots. (BYOTB*)

* Bring Your Own Tennis Ball

Ellie

Do you remember when we walked to the school before your Cross-Country meets? We always got there early before the bus or any of the other kids got there, and we walked a few laps around the track.

I remember how quiet and calm those early mornings were, before all the excitement and craziness of the races. You were so fast, and everyone had such high expectations of you. We watched your times so closely and discussed the upcoming course layouts and possible strategy, besides the usual, "Run till you puke!"

I hope you remember the most important message I had for you on those morning walks.

"Even if you trip at the start line and come in dead last, I will still love you just the same."

I always wanted you to know that I love you unconditionally. And I always will. You are a great person and I love you for who you are. Not for how many races you won or the choices you have ever made.

I want to reemphasize that because I don't think you ever got the message. I don't think you've ever failed at anything you put your mind to. When you graduated in December,

I was so curious what you were going to do, not worried, just curious. Your options were so wide open. The idea that you found something so perfect for you, so quickly, is unbelievable. You are truly making a difference in peoples' lives, whether you think you're getting through or not. And your office is beautiful.

I also am so happy with the friends you've made along the way. And how you don't let distance get in between you. You are a true friend, and they are a great support system when you need advice, a shoulder to cry on, or just tacos.

I love you. I hope you know that could never change. But I am also so proud of the young woman you have grown into.

Emily

You were my star show loving, hiking buddy when you were little and grew into my best movie watching partner,

I'm so happy I had those afternoons off when Ellie was in kindergarten and mom was working mornings. We had such a good time together going to the nature center in Bay and collecting our star show stamps. When I was doing in-center dialysis, the social worker had ways to settle my anxiety by leaving that place in my mind and going somewhere else that made me relax. Those surrounding trails with you is where I often found myself going back to.

I have so many fond memories of hanging out with you and our favorite movies always remind me of those times.

I'll never watch Dawn of the Dead without thinking of you whisper shouting "Dad, be quiet!" when I couldn't get my smuggled candy open, and I was disturbing the theater. I can't imagine The Sixth Sence without thinking of cuddling with you, watching on the ten-inch tablet. And don't even get me started on our favorite Quinton Tarantino films!? Watching Kill Bill takes on a whole new meaning when you watch it with a middle school girl. I don't know which one of us idolizes Beatrix Kiddo more.

As I'm writing this, you returned from studying abroad a month ago. I'm so glad you got to experience that. I tell people that you have done more during this semester than I've done in my whole life, and that's not an exaggeration. All the places you got to see, cultures you got to witness, and people you got to meet! You made the most of every minute and I'm so happy for you. I also appreciate you having fun stories from your different adventures, instead of the usual response of, "It was fine," with a shrug of the shoulders.

I'm excited to see where your life takes you when you finish school. You have the ability and work ethic to be anything you want. I just know you're going to do great things.

Thank you for visiting and taking interest in my dialysis machine. I thought about what you said about making a video showing how I set it up every day. I think I'm going to work on that next. That is if you'll help me with it, of course.

You are the only reason my first book exists. You dragged me, kicking and screaming, through that entire process. Never think that I don't appreciate your hard work, no matter how busy you were. I swear you have found a way to squeeze twenty-eight hours out of a normal day.

I love you and I'm proud of you every day.

Nate

I loved the days spent in your first and second grade classrooms. Reading to and helping you and your friends with math. It was as good for me as it ever was for your teacher. The best part was eating lunch together and walking home. It was only a mile or so, but it gave us time to really connect. I looked forward, all week, to those afternoons and your creative stories. Everyone says it because it's true, your kids grow up so fast. It seems like only last year we were camping with the Cub Scouts and now you are taking a two-week canoe trip where you are going to be one of the responsible ones.

I'm glad you have stuck with Scouts as long as you have, and it looks like you'll be earning your Eagle rank. This is no small task and I'm extremely proud of you for this achievement.

High school is so very different today than it was when I graduated. You seem to be doing well with everything, considering the many challenges you face. I'm glad Cross Country has been treating you well and that you are staying fit and having fun. (Thank you, Coach D, for looking out for him.)

I also love that, as busy as you are, we still find time to watch our Marvel movies together. I have always said that I appreciate movies more, because I can watch them through the eyes of a teenage boy. I enjoy your reactions as much, or more, than the movies themselves. Do you remember our shared excitement at Bruce Campbell's cameo in Dr. Strange!? That was amazing and something your two sisters would never understand.

Right now, you are playing Magic the Gathering and gaming on your new computer. I'm very curious if these interests will stick or if you will move on to other things. I know I still love the things I did at your age. As your grandpa says, "It's the best time of your life and no one ever tells you!"

I know we don't spend as much time together as we used to. For so many reasons, but this is supposed to be the time when you find friends and move on to bigger and better things. Just know that I love you more every day and I'm even more thankful for the times we do get together.

I love you and I'm proud of you and I think about you every day.

June 18

I started this nightly journal to coincide with my walking challenge for The National Kidney Foundation. walk thirty-three miles in thirty days to bring awareness to the thirty-three percent of people affected by chronic kidney disease.

Originally, I was going to log each day's mileage along with my month to date total at the bottom of each page. I found that to be rather redundant as I'm walking one mile every day and ya'll know how to keep adding one up to thirty, with a little bit extra on a few days towards the end.

When I was online, registering for the event, I somehow also registered for an in-person walk at the Science Center, in downtown Cleveland.

This was a three-mile walk, which I would double dip and count towards my monthly total. My worry was that I had done charity events in the past (See my MS ride in the Eight of Diamonds story.) and always had difficulty raising the expected donations. Everyone else seemed to ask so casually and the donations flowed in. While I was barely scraping by with a last-minute donation from "anonymous donor." I could only guess that was our team leader who didn't want his team members to make him look bad.

Now I had mistakenly posted two fundraisers for the same organization, each with its own insurmountable goal.

To my surprise my friends and family came through in a big way. I met both of my goals on the very first night, without doing anything besides posting them on Facebook. That meant so much to me. If you are one of the people who made such a generous donation, I thank you from the bottom of my heart. Together we raised over six hundred dollars for my in-person walk and we are already over our goal for the month-long challenge with almost two more weeks to go. As you've seen in the pages of this book, this cause and organization both mean so much to me, personally.

Now that the money was raised, I just had to do the walk. The first issue was that it was at 8:30 in Cleveland, an hour away from my parents' house. This was the earliest I had to wake up since I'd stopped working in November. Which is a problem because I'm stuck on the dialysis machine for eleven hours each night. If I had to wake up at seven and be out the door by seven thirty, that meant I had to be upstairs, in my bedroom, hooked up at eight the night before. This is why I've been hesitant to find another regular job. I had trouble waking up in the mornings before this and it had only gotten worse. It has been motivating me to write each night for this project however, since I'm stuck here for so long anyway.

I never sleep very well and last night was no different. I was up and preparing an hour before my alarm went off. I found some markers and my blank "I'm Walking For..." bib they had sent me.

"ASK ME ABOUT PD!" I wrote in my neatest capital block letters. Sure, it was tacky. But I thought it was better than "**MYSELF!**" and I have recently become an unofficial advocate for PD dialysis. I have been feeling great, living my life, and I wasn't afraid to tell anyone who was unsure about making the jump from the hell that was in-center.

Of course, I am just a patient with no skin in the game. And a patient who doesn't really understand the numbers all that well. I appreciate the smiley and frown faces throughout the report to tell me when I'm doing good and what I need to work on. (I know, Dr. Lee, take my binders! I got that much.) But I do think patients who aren't sure what they are getting into, and are nervous to hook up by themselves, my real-world experiences can help them make a more educated decision.

The walk was so much fun. It was a short, .2-mile loop around the parking lot. The DJ counted out the fifteen laps as the leaders came around each time. Each lap was dedicated to someone who had connections to chronic kidney disease. One for the donors, one for the recipients, a silent lap for those we've lost (I'll say I teared up during that one,) etc.

There were so many families and teams who came together to support their loved ones, it was really touching. Next year, I plan to be ready earlier and invite others to join me. So, start thinking of a team name now...

Also, and I can't explain where my recent love for dogs has come from, but there were so many sweet, well-behaved dogs walking with their owners. I couldn't help but think about how crazy Merida* is. As much as I love her, there would be no way she'd be able to attend an event like that without losing her fool mind.

I did make sure to stop at my house to scratch her

stomach, cuddle, and take a nap on the couch before driving back down to Wooster for the night.

*Merida is my poodle.

June 19

Today was Father's Day. It was the best one I ever had.

I met the kids in Strongsville, which is about halfway between our house in North Olmsted and my parents' in Wooter. We saw the early bird show of the Bob's Burgers Movie. It was pretty good, not my first pick but Ellie loves it and we had been wanting to see it since we first saw the trailers. I'll go see Buzz Lightyear by myself later this week.

After the movie, Jeanette met us for lunch at a fancy taco place. They got me chocolate covered grapes from Malley's which I've always wanted to try, a cool dinosaur, and a card with a Papasaur on it.

Nate had to get to work, so he went with Jeanette back home, but the girls wanted to go back to the mall to go shopping. This is normally where I would have declined and driven back to Wooster. But I still needed to get my mile walk in for the day and thought it would be nice to spend the afternoon with them.

We had a great time going into many different stores. We alternated between girly clothes stores and nerdy collectable stores. It was difficult, but I refrained from buying the Skeletor and Garbage Pail Kid, Adam Bomb, shirt. They were BıGı fifty percent off! (The verdict is still out; I might go back.)

I've mentioned not taking things for granted, and I think about how different the day would have been if I didn't feel as good as I do now, or worse. Jeanette and I have a friend from high school who lost her husband this past year. She posted a very touching collection of pictures in remembrance of him. In fact, I noticed a lot of Happy Heavenly Father's Day posts and I'm thankful that my family isn't going through that.

I'm really not trying to exaggerate the situation, but again, it's hard not to when I've seen so many people in similar situations pass away. I've seen so many stories on Facebook from caregivers and loved ones who have lost people close to them to kidney disease. And that name, "End Stage Kidney Failure" has such a sense of finality to it.

After laps on both floors of the mall, we stopped at the pet store and ogled over the puppies for a while, discussing how happy Jeanette would be if we surprised her with one, or all of them.

We made one last stop at the arcade for some Mario Kart. Ellie beat me, even though it is Father's Day, and she had no remorse about it either. (She gets her competitive nature from her mom.)

She drove me back across the street to my car, and we said our goodbyes. I drove home, stopping at the gas station on the way for my dad's present of beer. (All he ever gets is beer.) It had one of the Greek Gods on it and he said it was pretty good.

I shared some of my Malley's grapes with my mom and was glad they didn't melt into a giant chocolatey mess in the car.

Then, I crashed into my recliner. I don't have any plans until 2:00 tomorrow afternoon and I'm probably going to sleep in until about noon. I knew I might be overdoing it and I'm going to pay for it tomorrow. But it was absolutely worth it.

June 20

I know I have made this journey out to be all sunshine and butterflies. Probably read today's entry before you run out and sell both kidneys on the black market. (But if you still want to, I'll take one.)

There are bad days. There are mornings when I wake up exhausted. Whether it's because the dialysis machine was sassy, sounding it's alarm every hour or bad thoughts crept into my head at two in the morning and wouldn't leave. I played a few levels of Plants Vs Zombies, then checked Facebook. At this time, there usually isn't anything new, but you know how you can get to scrolling.

This morning there was a post from someone in one of the kidney groups I follow. They had been posting recently that they didn't know if it was worth it to keep going. Last night they decided it wasn't and they said a heartfelt goodbye, thanking the group as a whole for helping get as far as they did. They wished everyone well and said they would not be back. This was followed by lots of replies, mostly thoughts and prayers or "Talk to somebody."

I refrained from adding to the noise. I didn't have anything to say that someone else hadn't already said better. You'll never see me offering thoughts and prayers. And I have to resist offering my personal phone number to everyone on the internet. While I wish I could, I lack the time and, more importantly, the knowledge involved with handling these situations.

So, I did what anyone with depression and anxiety does in the middle of the night...

I logged onto Google and searched for suicide rates among dialysis patients. One study I found, from 2005, said that there were 24.2 suicide deaths per 100,000 dialysis patients. An 84% increase in risk over the general population. One third of these deaths occurred during the first three months on dialysis and half during the first year.

As I write this, I'm seven months and two weeks in. I haven't missed a session and I'm doing okay. Sometimes, I think back and I'm relieved that I was simply too exhausted to act on some of my impulses. I didn't see, but I will make an educated guess that a large percentage of these suicides take place late at night. Many of the dialysis patients I have met complain about insomnia. The loneliness can be soul crushing.

Even if things aren't nearly that bad for me, as I said before, there are bad days. I'd say after two or three days of relatively normal productivity, like waking up at a reasonable hour, driving an hour to Cleveland for a doctor or physical therapy appointment, spending some time at the house with my family, doing my daily walk, and driving back to my parents' house, I am usually drained the next day and find myself staying in bed, or my recliner, sleeping until two or three in the afternoon.

I used to beat myself up for this waste of time, but I have learned to accept it and plan for it.

One thing I've learned from the DaVita support group I'm in is that I'm not alone in this perpetual state of exhaustion. We all handle these days differently and we do the best we know how.

Just know that we aren't lazy, we are sick and we are tired and everyday we are trying to stay positive knowing that we made it through another long, sleepless night.

Update: Many concerned posts asked for a response from that man after not seeing any posts from him for a few days. He reassured the group that he was doing okay, and we were all relieved. It was nice to see everyone come together with concern for one of our members, one of our friends. He promised to continue posting.

June 21

We were moving into a new apartment in Olmsted Falls, this was before Nate, about '03 or '04. I had a parking lot full of friends helping us move in. It was a third-floor apartment with no elevator, and we were all standing around a pickup truck, debating the best way to get a heavy dresser out of the truck bed and up all those stairs. It was far too heavy for any one of us, but too small for any two of us to work together. My dad, Rick, came outside from his two-hundredth trip, with no shirt, he backed up to the rear of the pickup.

"Just push it onto my back" He wasn't asking, he was telling. He had seen us from the window and was tired of us wasting time.

"Dad, this thing is over a hundred pounds. You can't carry it alone."

"Well, you sissies don't seem to be making much progress with it. Let's get it done."

And so, two of us got into the truck and pushed it off the bed and onto his spine. He took a few steps to get his balance and he was off, up all three flights without a break to catch his breath. He left a group of ten men, standing awestruck, scrambling to grab boxes of clothes or pillows or anything to not let this man who was about thirty years older than most of us make them look bad.

My friends who witnessed this will never forget it and bring it up often. "Dude, remember that time when your dad..."

I tell that story because that has always been how my dad was. And still is. He was always there to help when we needed him, but he also didn't have the patience for bullshit. I think he would rather have my friends not been there, it would have meant more pizza and beer for him and I'm sure he thought he could have done it faster without them.

When I was a kid, my dad gave me a twenty dollar bill to go up to Dairy Mart at the corner to buy some snacks and rent a movie. Of course, I lost the twenty, didn't get anything after the three mile walk, and didn't have his change. I don't remember him even getting mad and he didn't even make me pay that money back. He just wanted me to let my little brother hang out with us in our tent that night in the backyard.

I could fill this entire book with stories about how badass my dad is, but I realize I almost did with my last book. (See 7 of Spades, King of Diamonds, 4 of Clubs) Today I want to thank him. He literally saved my life by taking me in in November and doesn't even make a big deal about it. This disease has turned my life upside down, and he has had to make just as many adjustments to his own life.

I don't remember asking, or if it was just accepted, but I

went home with them when I was released from the hospital. Jeanette is working full time at a new job that she loves and I was too weak to walk without help or drive. He was going to drive me to and from dialysis for all of my sessions as well as take me up to my doctor's visits in Cleveland, of which there were many, smooshed into every Tuesday and Thursday as those were the only two days I was free from those machines.

There were a lot of snowy mornings, when he was outside at seven, shoveling the long driveway, to get us out on time. I'm sure he would have loved to sit inside with his coffee, watching the snow fall. I didn't miss a single treatment. He'd wait outside when he was able. It was the peak of Covid, after all. But often the nurses ran outside to get him when I was in bad shape. He'd convince them I was okay when I got home, ate something, and took a nap. He would carry my frail, puking, body out to the car. We had a system worked out. He kept garbage bags and paper towels in the back seat and we usually stopped at Jimmy John's on the way home. The basic turkey sandwich was one of two things I could keep down.

The other is my dad's chili! And my dad made a lot of chili! No beans, light tomatoes, no spices. He added most of that to his own after scooping mine. It was just ground beef and a bunch of peppers. I was on a high protein diet for my bed sore to heal and this checked that box for sure.

He was nervous about me falling down the stairs, so we set up a makeshift, temporary bedroom in the dining room. I slept there for about four months and covered that table with all my crap. My parents essentially lost half of their main floor during that time.

Also, I was sleeping all the time. They didn't have to worry about waking me up. But I think they still felt bad making too much noise in the mornings.

I finally was able to drive on my off days, but he still had to take me to and from dialysis. He was great about working this new life around his schedule of hiking, Wal-Mart trips, and Chipotle. (It's true, nobody likes Chipotle more than Rick Templeton!) This went on until I was able to start PD.

PD brought on its own challenges. We keep the supplies in the basement, and he has to carry the heavy boxes of fluid up two flights of stairs, twice a week. He sometimes works this into his workout routine. But usually he also does his daily hike or lifts his weights.

I feel bad, because I think he sleeps very lightly since I've been staying with him. He is always ready to wash out a dirty bucket or run into my room when I knock my cycler to the floor at three in the morning.

"I don't want to touch it, it might break."

"Dad, I think that ship has sailed! You're going to have to touch it to pick it up!"

Now that we are talking about transplant, he is going to continue taking care of me for the four to six weeks of recovery. That will be a lot of me laying around and a lot of trips to Cleveland Clinic's Main Campus. He's not thrilled about driving downtown, but he also doesn't hesitate to do whatever it takes to help me out.

My dad taught me three valuable life lessons when I was little and they apply to everyone. I'm going to share them, today, with you.

1. Don't try to jump onto a moving train. It might look like it's going slow, but it's not. It'll suck your legs underneath and cut them off!

2. Never run over a bag with your car. Assume it's filled with nails and broken glass. It'll pop your tires!

3. The casinos on the Vegas strip aren't there because gamblers win. Everyone loses!

Okay, it's past 1:00 in the morning and I could honestly sing my dad's praises forever. I could also share hundreds of other useful advice my dad has given me over the years.

I'm going to wrap it up by saying that I love him for everything he has and continues to do for me, and beyond that, it has been great spending all this time together.

Also, he got me hooked on the Justified TV show. I can't thank him enough for that.

Also, also, he got air conditioning installed for the first time in his life and it is currently forty degrees in here.

June 22

Tonight, I want to talk about my beautiful wife, Jeanette. She has been such a rockstar through all of this. She has been working her job that she loves, taking care of the kids (and that dog), managing our finances, and redoing each room in the house. She really is amazing. I look forward to after transplant and recovery when I'm able to move back home. I'm sure Merida won't be happy about giving up my side of the bed.

She has been working her tail off lately and I hope she knows I appreciate her every day. One of the things we talk about in group is not assuming how other people feel. We need to communicate our feelings and have real discussions about what's going on. I have been trying, but I still wonder what she's going to think when she reads some of these chapters. I know I didn't express some of these feelings out loud to her. It's funny the things we are too afraid to tell the ones we love, but it's not so hard to type it out for the entire world to read.

I feel bad for what Jeanette has gone through lately. She was very close to her mom, who passed away two years ago after a long, hard battle with cancer. Jeanette stayed by her side until the end. It was very difficult then and it has not gotten any easier with time. Now I'm sick and she's really having a hard time with it. She's so worried about me, for good reason.

I try to do little things when I'm able to cheer her up. I was going to get her flowers and surprise her at her work, but a doctor's appointment went long, and I didn't have time to stop at the store. I showed up empty handed and explained my good intentions. (I know, fill one hand with good intentions and shit in the other and see which one fills up first.) I think she appreciated the gesture, and it was better than me showing up to her empty office with a dozen roses in my hand. I was also up in Cleveland this week and I surprised the family with dinner. It was great spending time with them, and I was able to use money I earned on a Papa visit, so it relieved a little bit of that burden for the week. It was nice to just spend a few hours with the family. I know it is how things have to be right now and I am able to accept it most of the time. But, some nights, I miss her so much. That's another one of those thoughts that sneak into my insomnia ridden head and won't go away.

I love Jeanette with all my heart...

...Can somebody let her know which page this is? I learned long ago that she hates to read, even if it's a book by her husband.

June 23

Earlier this month, I mentioned "the bad days." This is one of those days. I don't know if I've just been doing too much this week or if the heat has been getting too me. Either way, I don't have the energy to write how I'd like, and I don't have much to say...

That being said, I've kept this in my back pocket knowing this day would come.

This story is from my good friend, Mike. When I asked old GameStop co-workers for stories for my unpublished work stories book, he was the one who sent one in. I didn't want his time and efforts to go to waste.

Alright kids, behave for your substitute. I'll be back tomorrow.

Growing up I was never into roller coasters or amusement parks, in general. Growing up in northeast Ohio, I'd gone to Cedar Point as a kid with family, sure, but I only ever really rode Mine Ride or Avalanche Run (which was later turned into Disaster Transport), which were the tame coasters. I rode my first 'big' roller coaster when I was 19, in the summer of 2000: Raptor.

When I got off of Raptor, I was obsessed. I ended up going back to Cedar Point two more times that season and have had season passes every year since then.

By the year 2011, Cedar Point had gone through some changes, as parks do over time. Rides have been razed; some have been raised. But there was still one coaster that I just couldn't bring myself to ride and that fateful day in August, I finally had my chance.

When I began working at GameStop in 2010, I befriended my store manager, and you may have heard of him – Cal. He and I had many things in common, including our hobby of Cedar Point. With Cal being the store manager, and I being the Assistant Store Manager, it was very rare that both of us be off on the same day. Usually, we'd go hang out there, either just the two of us, or with his family, after work on a Saturday, even when we'd close at 9pm.

On Friday, August 5, 2011, the stars seemed to align perfectly. I remember it well. Cal was on vacation, or maybe he wasn't. Or maybe I was on vacation? Who knows! Either way, we were both out at the park. Cal brought the kids – or at least Nate – again, it's been ten years, and my brain is a bit foggy nowadays. Nate, being much younger, and smaller than he is today, 'cause that's how aging works, wasn't quite tall enough to ride the big, big rides, but enjoyed riding one roller coaster in particular, the one that I'd yet to ride myself – Keep in mind, that at this time I'd been to dozens of parks, 125 different roller coasters ridden – yet had not ridden this ONE roller coaster at Cedar Point, my own personal White Whale.

Yes, you guessed it: Jr. Gemini.

This coaster, built in 1979 was a steel behemoth, standing a whopping NINETEEN feet tall, and reached a maximum speed of SIX miles per hour. And yet, I had not ridden this.

"Why?" you may be asking yourself? Because to ride this particular coaster and you are over 54" tall, you must be accompanied by a child. Me, being six-foot-three, and not having a child of my own at the time, made things difficult to complete the list of Cedar Point coasters. Asking strangers to borrow their kids so I could ride was out of the question – I had watched friends do this in the past. It was cringe-worthy, yet hilarious.

So here I am, 30-years old, 6'-3", 280 lb me – convincing Nate to allow me to tag-along with him on his fifty second journey. I'm super excited at this point. We wait in line, which takes forever due to this ride only having one train, so it has to go around, twice, then unload, then load again. Rinse and repeat.

Finally, it is our turn. Nate wants the 5th car. We sit down. Pull the lap bar down – ah crap.

Did I mention I was 6'-3" tall? My knees are too tall for the "T" of the lap bar to come down over. I try crossing my legs, twisting and turning, bending things that could be bent like a discount contortionist. And frankly, I was putting on a free Coney Island freak show for those standing in line.

Somehow, finally, I manage to get my knee into a position in such a way that the lap bar came down to my hip and I was then able to bend my knee back up, around the end of the lap bar.

And we were off! Two laps around the 400' long track. Two times up the lift hill. Two times reaching that maximum velocity of 6mph. And it was rough. With how the restraint pinned me, I felt every nook and cranny that those wheels and track had endured since 1979 – the wheels were more than likely from 2011, but the track having been through the elements for 32 years, had seen better days.

Now, I know you aren't reading this book for the biology it exudes, but the human body isn't as rigid as a roller coaster car. The shakes and vibrations of the 50 second ride caused just enough movement that my body settled into the car, and slipped into a position that when we got back to the station to unload... I couldn't get out. The lap-bar, when rising, would hit my thigh and could not get over my knee. And with how I was positioned, I couldn't straighten my leg enough, or bend it around the restraint to get out.

For what seemed like an eternity, ride attendants were trying to get my legs free of the ride – again, there's awkward me, putting on a free David Copperfield escape act for the same people-- did I mention, this only had one train? – that saw me cram myself into this steel trap to begin with.

After about five minutes, I just said the heck with it, and summoned the power of Thor and finally squeezed my thunder thighs out of the ride, crushing my favorite pair of sunglasses, that were in my front pocket in the process. When I returned home and got ready for bed for the evening, I also found that I had a nice 6" bruise on my inner thigh from the ordeal.

So, thanks to Cal and I having simultaneous time off from work to go out to Cedar Point, I was able to rent a child in order to completely humiliate myself in front of strangers. It was well worth it.

June 24

It's not a kidney thing, but I have Macular degeneration in my eyes and since all these issues stem from my diabetes, we might as well talk about it.

It doesn't happen often but sometimes my eye will "fade out." It's difficult to explain. It starts with just a few tiny, black, squiggly lines in my vision. Then, usually by the end of the day, I can't see at all out of one eye. I'm usually able to avoid driving when it happens or at least, just short trips around the block, sticking to familiar roads. This started yesterday and I stayed inside and rested all day.

I haven't been to the eye doctor for over a year with everything else I've been dealing with. Also, the process of slowing down this issue is rather unpleasant. For anyone with a thing about eye stuff, this is your worst nightmare. What is actually happening is that the damaged blood cells in the back of the eyeball are getting stirred up and blocking my vision (Or so I'm told, Google it if you care to learn more. I'm not a doctor.) There is medicine that is injected into my eyes. And not near my eyes either. Directly into my eyeballs.

I don't know about their other patients, but they get frustrated when I tear up and blink.

"UGH! We've got a blinker. Get the shields!"

"Yeah, we can just skip the step where we try without the shields. I promise I'm going to blink every time you come at me with that damn needle."

In comes the assistant with these clear shields that tuck in under my eyelids. It holds them open, Clockwork Orange style, and they have a tiny hole in the center for the needle.

"Now you'll feel a little pinch."

SPLAT! It's hard to describe how gross it is when it actually happens. Go watch Zombie for the world's worst splinter (And a great shark vs. zombie fight!) or Brightburn. Or Demons. Or Final Destination 5. Or Kill Bill Volume 2. This list could go on for three pages. I'll stop here. If you've seen any of these movies, you remember those scenes well. If you haven't, you have some homework to do.

The last time I did this, they sent me out into the bright morning sunshine to drive back to work. I couldn't see anything and stumbled out to my car to wait for my vision to return.

These shots are supposed to be a temporary fix leading up to surgery where they use a laser to seal up the blood vessels. I've never made it that far in the process, but I have an appointment tomorrow where I will talk about that option.

The transplant doctors told me to not let this get away from me and I want to make sure I do everything I can not to jeopardize my chances to get on the list.

June 25

It worked out that this has been a good month to record my daily thoughts. I am doing better than I have since being diagnosed in early November. This week I will be going to the hospital twice to finish up my last few tests before they meet and decide whether I can be added to the transplant list. It makes sense, they don't want to give a kidney to someone without a strong enough heart to support it.

It's not a sure thing but all the doctors and my transplant coordinator seem to think I'm a good candidate.

I was asked a question in this week's DaVita support group that caught me off guard...

"What now? What are you going to do differently?"

I've been looking at life in the very short term. "End Stage" anything will do that to a person.

Now that a transplant is possibly in my future, (The wait is two to six years for a cadaver but much shorter with a live donor, which I have a few possibilities lined up.) I don't know what I'm going to do.

I think I'm going to travel a little. And swim. It's true that you "don't know what you got (till it's gone)" from Cinderella's hit ballad off their 1988 cassette, Long Cold Winter. I never cared to travel much, but now that I know I can't, I'm jealous of all the pictures my friends are posting on Facebook.

And swimming, I've never been one to swim. Now that I'm not allowed to swim, or my port will get infected, I miss being able to on these hundred-degree days.

I think I'll start in Colorado. It's been too long since I've been out to see my Aunt Vicky. She's in Fort Collins and it's so beautiful out there. Plus, it's not far from the Rocky Mountains and eight hours to Yellowstone. An eight-hour drive used to seem like forever to me, but recently, it doesn't seem so bad. Just the idea of flying has been so far off my radar with all the supplies I would need to have shipped and everything that could go wrong. (Do you get upset when they lose your luggage?)

Next, I might head out to an ocean. I didn't see the ocean until I was about thirty years old and that was only for five minutes when my friend, Richard, took me to see it. Then again when we went to the beach and the sand was hotter than hell and my daughter, Emily, and I got chased out of the water by jellyfish. I've always said I didn't need to go back, but maybe I'll give it another try.

I might not be ready to dance around my room, lip syncing to Timbuk 3's The Future's so Bright I Gotta Wear Shades, but I can at least start with my favorite Andy Grammer song, Good to Be Alive (Hallelujah).

June 26

The doctors weren't happy with my emergency chest catheter from the hospital. The preferred placement for a port is in the arm, called a fistula. They were concerned that mine would get infected and that the infection would go straight to my heart.

The one nice thing about hemodialysis is that the nurses do everything. You can just sit back while they clean the dressing and hook you into the machine. When they clean the site, they would tell me that it is slightly red and puffy.

"How long has it looked like this?"

"I have no idea." That was true. I was afraid to ever look at it and I never once removed the bandages to look underneath.

"Okay, let's keep an eye on it."

"I will." I absolutely would not be keeping an eye on it!

It is attached to a vein about where your collarbone is, and the tubes hang down about three inches to some clips that make hooking up easy for the nurses and they don't have to use needles at all.

The most important thing is that much like Gizmo, you absolutely cannot get it wet. This meant swimming was out, but more importantly, no more showers. I don't remember how it worked with baths. I might have been able to take baths if I kept it up and out of the water. But I was seeing a different doctor about the bedsore on my butt. She told me not to let it get submerged in water or that open wound would get infected.

So, for a few months after my hospital stay, I couldn't pee, couldn't shower or bathe, couldn't sit, and couldn't stand. And the bedsore was practically in my butt crack, so I had to be very careful whenever I pooped. But other than those few things, I was feeling fine.

My wife didn't fully understand that I wasn't allowed to shower and bought me some plastic covers to tape over the port when I would come home. I took it out of its packaging, and it was much smaller than we expected. I put it on the best I could, but only one side stuck properly. I called Jeanette in to show her, and together we opened another of these big stickers and overlapped to get coverage on the other side. And another one to hold the bottom in place. These were not cheap, and we were blowing through the entire package on the first day. She slapped some medical tape over the edges for good measure and into the shower I went.

It had been a month of sanitary wipes and I was excited to really wash the accumulated grime off of me. I don't know if it was the heat or the water, or the combination of both, but our cover immediately shriveled up and fell into the tub. As happy as I was to take a shower again, I hurried along, thinking of dying from a heart infection the entire time.

I hopped out of the shower and dried off really well with multiple towels. I didn't take many showers over the following six months. The reward wasn't worth the risk.

When I switched over to PD, the thing I looked most forward to was getting rid of that chest catheter and taking a true shower again.

Once you have the surgery, you have to wait a few weeks for it to heal before you can use it. Then, there is also a two-week training stage to make sure it's working correctly. For that month, I had both the tube coming out of my stomach and the port in my chest. With all this hardware, I felt like I was halfway to becoming the next Darth Vader (Or *Tetsou: The Iron Man*, but that's a deep cut reference that only true horror movie fans will know.)

Finally, I had been doing PD at home for a few weeks and I brought a day's worth of pee into the lab along with the drainage bags of all my belly juices. Sherry had it all tested to make sure it was pulling out all the toxins it was supposed to and after we made some tweaks to my nightly treatments, she scheduled a surgery to have my chest catheter removed.

It only took a few minutes. After I got the bill, my dad's joke of him pulling it out with a wrench didn't sound so bad. It actually took longer for the nurse to stand over me putting pressure on the site to wait for it to stop bleeding. Once it did stop, she covered it with a small bandage, told me to wait a day or two for a scab to form, then I'd be able to shower to my heart's content.

Those next two days were the longest two days of my life. And two nights later, I packed all my clean clothes and fresh bandages for my new belly PD port and went down to the basement shower at my parents.

I spent longer in that shower than any teenage boy ever

has. I turned that hot water all the way up and let it rinse off six months of crud.

If John Rambo had the worst shower in First Blood, then this would rank up there among the best. I think if I had to, I would have let them blast me with the hose.

When I was done, I followed the directions for drying off to keep my new port from getting infected. I use a lot of clean towels now whenever I have to shower.

I paused to look in the mirror before putting on my fresh t-shirt. I looked over my new scar on my shoulder and knew what it represented, the worst four months of my life. That's my version of a tattoo, along with all the scars from the holes they punched in my stomach to insert my PD port. They mean more to me than any art that I would choose for myself. They are constant reminders of what I've been through.

June 27

Years ago, when internet gaming was still in its infancy, I was excited at the prospect of playing chess online.

"Hello." I typed into the chat as I moved my king pawn forward two spaces. Nate makes fun of me because I always open with my king pawn.

"ASL"

"I'm sorry, I don't know what that means." I replied.

"Age, Sex, Location!?" The other player clarified. They still hadn't made their first move.

"Oh, sorry. 32, Male, Cleveland, Ohio."

YOU WIN!
COMPETITOR TERMINATED CONNECTION!
FIND A NEW GAME?
YES/NO

Oh well. I moved the curser over to YES. the 56K modem, beeped back at me as it thought. The screen flashed and the pawn reset back to its original position.

"Hello." I said as I moved the pawn forward again.

"ASL?"

Ugh, "32, Male, Cleveland, Ohio" I entered again.

YOU WIN!
COMPETITOR TERMINATED CONNECTION!
FIND A NEW GAME?
YES/NO

And that was the end of that. I didn't try playing online chess again for the next twelve years. I just didn't understand who these guys thought they were going to meet on a chess website. Would they have kept playing if I was a "18, Female, Miami, Florida?"

I think about those two single move chess games while I'm reading Facebook posts about people who are about to go on dialysis and are confused and scared. I want to offer help even though I have only been doing it for less than a year, I already have so much built-up knowledge (Like enough to fill up a small book!) I tread very lightly, however. The last thing they need is for me to come off as some type of creeper. Do people have no shame that hitting on vulnerable women on the verge of dialysis is a thing? It's also often wives who are on Facebook looking for advice because their husbands are too bullheaded to consider doing dialysis. "Sure, your husband is dying, and you're upset and want to help him. why don't you give me a call and we'll talk about it?" Tell me how to express that without coming off like a true scumbag.

Some days I find myself texting and calling five people within a few hours. I don't know why, but I'm really passion-ate about PD dialysis and there is so little information available about it. Honestly, I would have been nervous too, if I had the chance to think about it. As I said I had to get off hemodialysis and was going to do anything to do it. It wasn't until I was a week into training that I got really nervous about whether I could do it or not. And by then, I had the surgery and a tube coming out of my belly. There was no turning back, no matter how much doubt I had.

I talked to a man in Texas this evening for about forty minutes. He hadn't started dialysis yet and said it was really important that he could continue working. I explained everything to the best of my knowledge but reminded him that I'm not a doctor and these are just my experiences. I wished him luck and I think he really appreciated a patient's point of view on everything. It's kind of interesting how I can talk to a complete stranger about stool softeners and my nightly bathroom habits.

The opposite end of the spectrum was when I was texting back and forth with a young man (based on his profile picture.) He was meeting with his doctor to discuss options for his inevitable, upcoming dialysis. I gave him a little information through text, but he didn't want to talk on the phone. I checked up on him a few days after his appointment and asked him which way he decided to go.

"Neither. I like my life and I think I'd rather die than go on dialysis." he typed back.

This broke my heart and reminded me that this wasn't as easy as I thought it would be. I'm not a doctor and certainly not a therapist or social worker. I told him that I am getting back to my life and that I'm sure his friends and family wouldn't agree with his decision. We stopped talking after that, but I was glad to see he was back on Facebook, saying he had decided on PD. He wasn't happy about it, but willing to give it a chance. I hope that talking with me helped him make a good decision that will work for him.

I am starting my training next week to become a mentor for The National Kidney Foundation. I will talk with people who are new to dialysis and hopefully I will be able to help people who are just as scared as I was when this all started for me. The virtual groups that I'm in have helped me so much and I'd like to see patients get the support they need to not feel so alone in their battle against this scary disease.

If you are reading this and having a hard time, please talk to someone. Hell, as long as you don't expect any real medical advice, feel free to call or text me anytime at 440-502-0980.

June 28

If there is any silver lining to this whole kidney disease situation, it's that I've been able to spend the last six months with my mom. Like so many other families, we missed out on so much time over the last couple of years due to COVID restrictions. We skipped so many holidays and birthdays and visits in general. Now that I'm living with them, we've been able to make up for that lost time.

My parents live such a relaxing, laid-back lifestyle. There's nothing they love more than sitting out in the garage, watching the birds and chipmunks outside, and listen to their new CD's they bought at garage sales that week.

I spent so many years working in retail that it is so refreshing to see my parents who don't care about the newest, most expensive phone. They don't have Wi-Fi or a computer, and, most importantly, they don't miss these things. They have plenty of CDs and DVDs to keep them entertained forever and if they ever do need more, they can always find something at the next street sale.

My mom and I worked on converting my grandma's poetry into a small book. That was such a fun project, and it came out really well. It was neat to read through all of her old journals and it gave me a sense of where my mom got her life-long love of reading and writing. That same love wore off on me as well. I'm glad she raised me with a never-ending supply of great books. I swear, growing up, our basement had more books than the local library. I was never at a loss when it was time for a book report.

My mom wrote a column for the local paper and also ran the Maple Press, my elementary school's monthly paper. I was really proud in the sixth grade when they had a "celebrity" come in and speak to the English class. Of course, it was my mom, and all the other kids were impressed that she was so famous.

In a world of so much fighting and hate, I give my mom credit for raising me right. She taught me the golden rule of always treating others the way I wished to be treated. More importantly, she was never a hypocrite. She lives everyday of her life like that.

She is also the one who taught me to love family uncon-ditionally. When my brothers or I used to get in trouble, and with three boys, there was plenty of trouble, she always let us know it was okay.

"I love you more than I could ever love that dish you broke." Was just an example of how she looked at things.

Also, my mom has been taking care of my dad for over forty years. That alone makes her eligible for sainthood.

Not that it needs to be said, but I love my mom more every day.

June 29

I started this project, and stayed motivated throughout, because of The National Kidney Foundation 33-Mile Challenge. I'm happy to say I met or exceeded all of my goals that I set before this started.

First, I raised a decent amount of money for the cause. Thank you to my Facebook friends who made that happen on the very first night I shared the donation link. This book would have been very difficult to work on if I was stressing over finding donations at the same time.

Second, I went to the other Kidney Foundation walk downtown, earlier in the month. I walked two of the three miles that day, but just getting out of bed to get there in time was a huge victory for me.

Third, I kept up my average of a mile per day, plus a little more. It was really hot a few days, so I skipped, but I planned ahead for those days and banked a few extra miles when I was feeling pretty good.

Finally, the goal I had set at the beginning of this journey was to walk the entire 1.75-mile loop at Oak Hill in Wooster, Ohio. The paved path is marked every .25 and I started in the middle of May, going to the first mark and back, alternating direction each day. After a week, I started making it to the .5 marks and then back for an even mile. Then .75 for a mile and a half. Then, I decided to go for the whole loop. That first time all the way around was very difficult. An old couple saw me and were truly concerned as to whether I'd make it back up the hill to the parking lot. Spoiler: I did.

I wouldn't have even attempted this and certainly wouldn't have succeeded without Amanda's help. She's my physical therapist and has been working with me since April. What a difference two months can make.

My first visit was mostly tests to see what I was able to do. Which wasn't much. She also asked me about my history and goals. She watched me walk and suggested some leg braces on Amazon. They were affordable and while they might not have been the perfect solution for my weak ankles and foot fall, "I would actually wear them." That was important since I had these terrible braces before that didn't fit right and dug into my shins. They weren't doing me any good sitting at home in the closet. I've worn those braces every day since I got them.

Amanda gives me new workouts to do each week. It's funny how easy these look when she shows me the example.

"Stand with your feet together... Okay, now close your eyes."

"Yeah, this is dumb." Whoops, as I start to topple over and she catches me. Maybe that giant fashionable support strap isn't dumb after all.

I think the most important part of seeing her was talking out my feelings towards my walker. She understood how I didn't like using it, but she laid out my two choices. I could use it on my long walks or I could just not walk and spend all my time in my recliner at home. She knew I had spent the majority of the last five months in that chair and I was ready to get moving again. It was time for me to put aside the stigma and embarrassment of being the guy with a walker and embrace it.

Amanda knew my limits and how to push them a little further each week. She knows when I need a pat on the back for a job well done or a quick tap on my shoulder to remind me to relax them. (Always, they are always too tense.)

If there is any one person directly responsible for keeping me walking throughout this challenge, which is also what has kept me writing, it is Amanda.

June 30

There it is. A month in the life of a dialysis patient. If you're still reading, I thank you for sticking with me till the end.

Was it what you expected? Probably not. Was it the only thing I could bring myself to write? Absolutely. I hope I did okay explaining how this disease affects the body, but just as much, or more, the mind.

I'm sorry if I rambled at points and I'm sorry if this made you uncomfortable. I tried to keep it light, but some of these topics are pretty heavy.

I wrote most of this with my dialysis family in mind. And those who are unfortunate enough to join our tight knit community, either as a patient, a family member, or a caregiver.

I've only been fighting this fight for seven months, but it seems like much longer than that. I'm in a good place now and always moving forward.

I appreciate the love and patience everyone has shown me while I worked to get to where I am now. I'm going to keep fighting and hope you find the strength and courage to as well. Whether it's dialysis or your own personal struggle. I wish you well.

And I promise I'll be in a better place next time and I won't be such a Debbie Downer.

Love, Cal

Acknowledgements

Thank you to Amanda (relax your shoulders) Guberinic, my physical therapist. I couldn't imagine walking these miles a few months ago.

Thank you to Lori, Kyra, Allison, Molly, and Suzanne, my social workers at DaVita. You were there for me during my hardest times. I will never forget the compassion and empathy you showed me, when I needed it most.

Thank you to my friends who didn't let the long drive stop you from seeing me when I really needed visitors. Also, everyone who came to see me in the hospital. I know it was a pain in the butt to schedule with COVID protocols and visitor restrictions.

Thanks to all my nurses and doctors I've seen along this journey. I know I haven't always been the easiest patient to work with. Sherry, my PD nurse. You are amazing and have taught me well.

Thank you to my family. This book took a lot of time and energy and I appreciate your patience and understanding as I worked through it.

Kenny Peris, thank you for another great cover. You are always a class act, and you know how to put my ridiculous ideas to paper.

Mike McCormack, thank you for providing that story and giving me a day off.

Steve "With the Hat" Schuerger, your generosity towards my family, during our time of need will never be forgotten.

Aunt Vicky, you are the kindest and most genuine person I have ever met. You are a wonderful role model for my daughters to look up to. Thank you for everything. I love you.

Thank you, Emily, again you get half the credit for getting this into people's hands. Writing it all is only half the job - honestly, it's the easy half.

Thank you to my mom and dad. You are wonderful hosts.

Finally, thank you, Steve Glick. You were there at the hospital within the first few days offering to help with the most generous gift imaginable. You are the best friend a guy could ever ask for.

About the Author

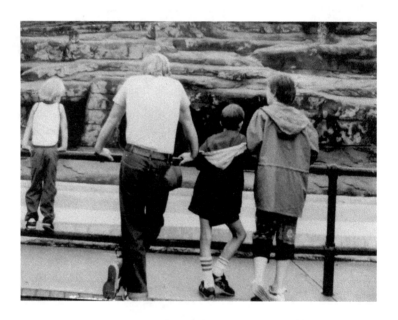

One time, he went to the zoo with his family.

Also Available

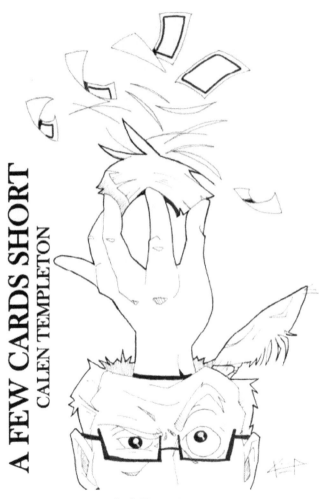

A FEW CARDS SHORT

CALEN TEMPLETON

Get It Now at Amazon.com

CPSIA information can be obtained
at www.ICGtesting.com
Printed in the USA
BVHW031040200722
642186BV00009B/35